"HEAVENLY BEING"

"HEAVENLY BEING"

A witness to glorious life after death

JOE DAVID WREN

MCP BOOKS

MCP Books
2301 Lucien Way #415
Maitland, FL 32751
407·339·4217
www.MCPBooks.com

Unless otherwise indicated, Scripture quotations taken from the King
James Version (KJV)–*public domain*.

Printed in the United States of America.

ISBN-13: 9781545614228

Contents

SEPTEMBER 2, 2016. "YELL OUT, 9-1-1!" WAS THE utterly unmistakable shout I heard. Yet, miraculously, it hadn't come from any earthly being. This heartfelt and solemn warning came as a direct gift from the Lord Almighty through the Holy Ghost. No Earthly being would have or could have gained my absolute and immediate attention, even as I precariously hovered in such a cadaverous condition. In fact, though dying, my body felt consumed by the Holy Spirit, making it so undeniably clear, even in those final seconds before death, that I heard, listened, and obeyed.

"CALL 9-1-1" were my final words, projected just one second after receiving that heaven-sent prompting. From there, I was finished. I vaguely remember my knees buckling, but in the very short time it took for me to fall to the ground, I became fully unconscious.

Chapter 1:

A New Home

September 1, 1966

A S I WATCHED THE RICKETY, TARNISHED YELLOW school bus pull to a stop on Commercial Avenue in Anaconda, Montana, my heart raced. I was six years old, alone in a new town, preparing for my first day of school at George Washington Elementary, and I was very scared.

It was early in the fall of 1966, and not only was the nation deeply involved in the Vietnam War, so was my heroic father. While I was entirely unaware of it at the time, at that very moment, somewhere in the jungles of Southeast Asia, Dad was battling his way to Purple Hearts and multiple Medals of Valor via war battles so vicious that most Americans dared not even think about them. His only prominent praise came from the highest office in the nation when President John F. Kennedy personally awarded him a commemorative plaque for being a part of our nation's first group of elite Green Beret Special Forces.

Yet there I was, boarding my first school bus with knees shaking so hard I stumbled as I attempted to climb in.

While the horrors of war didn't take my dad's life physically, emotionally and spiritually they took a major toll on him, his marriage, and his family. My young mother, Barbara, herself battling depression from the consequential effects of fear, sadness, and loneliness brought on by combat, had filed for divorce that summer and anxiously awaited one of Dad's few breaks from war to tell him. His continuous and harrowing duties of perilous fighting missions in that foreign land sometimes kept

1

him away from our family for many months at a time. Though she loved her husband, the challenges of watching him return from abominable Delta Project battles had increasingly become too heavy for her to bear.

Finally the day came when she would inform Dad face-to-face that she was moving my brothers, Mike and Bob, and me with her across the country from Ft. Bragg, North Carolina, to a small town in southwest Montana in search of a new start. My heroic father, who had patriotically and courageously risked his life time after time for his country, fell to his knees sobbing on the tarmac as he helplessly and hopelessly watched our plane take off.

The realization that he'd just lost his family had sunk in for him, and the awful pain of us leaving my father, as well as the deep emotional scars on my heart, would take decades to overcome. Only the Lord's hand itself could ever save my family.

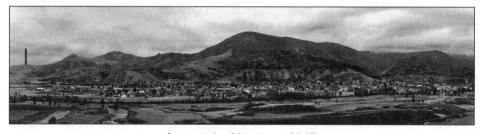

Anaconda, Montana 2017

Anaconda was a nationally prominent mining town back in the mid-1960s. I loved it then, and I love it now. This historic and visually stunning area continues to be made up of hard-working, wonderful, and proud people. It is also home to one of the world's largest smokestacks, once run by miners who were known to work hard and play harder. At one time, Anaconda was said to have more bars per square mile than any other town in America. As I climbed aboard the loud and raucous school bus on that chilly September morning, I witnessed that wild smelter-city parental exuberance that was clearly handed down to their youth.

Mom worked hard each day—she had to. Being a single parent in the 1960s with three young boys required two full-time

2

jobs. Job one was to make money, and job two was to make sure her young boys would one day turn into fine young men. So we moved into a very inexpensive fourplex apartment and began adjusting as quickly as we could.

"Well, are you going to come in or *walk* to school, kid?" roared the aging driver as I stood staring incredulously up into the school bus. "I ain't got all day!" Meekly making my way aboard, I skirted past him, taking time to note the rugged, crevice-filled face of this poor, child-weary driver. His years of shepherding boisterously loud schoolkids had clearly taken a physical toll, forcing me to at least consider the merits of a brisk walk instead. As I silently walked down the aisle between the seats, I asked God to bless me with some like-minded friend to sit beside. Though I'd rarely even been inside a church at the time, somehow—inherently—I always knew God lived, that He loved me, and that He was one I could count on at any critical moment.

Making my way down that inharmonious gauntlet of stares, shoves, and flying paper airplanes, I eventually spotted an open seat next to a scruffy young first-grader named Tracy Moses. Instantly I surmised him as a combination of Charlie Brown and Huckleberry Finn—two of my favorites. "Okay if I sit by ya?" I meekly asked. "I guess," he answered in a less-than-cheerful tone. Tracy may not have been the best-dressed or most popular kid on the block, but neither was I. That turned out to be reason enough that, from that moment on, Tracy became my dear friend—for life, as it turned out. I guess you could say that back then we *both* lived on the wrong side of the tracks. Rarely did either of us have a nickel to our name— and when we did, it would almost immediately be cashed in at the Dairy Queen for a small ice cream cone. But we did hold on to our pride, enthusiasm, and what dignity we could muster. From that day on, Tracy and I kindled a friendship that would last decades. What began shortly before man first walked on the moon would become a giant step for me as I learned to negotiate life without a father to lead and guide me—at least not an earthly father.

The months and years ahead would constantly provide challenging opportunities for growth. Mom's paycheck, like that

3

of virtually every other underpaid woman at the time, barely covered the basics. While we had ample food and shelter, her entertainment account was generally empty, except for allowing us an occasional visit to the twenty-five-cent matinee at the local Washoe Theatre. In those days, the theater would often be so filled with miners' children that owner Henry Lussey would take the stage prior to the opening credits and instruct us that we'd have to sit two kids to a seat to fit every child in! None of us complained, because it was still the highlight of the week, and that minor inconvenience only seemed to add to our fun. Today the Washoe Theatre is proudly listed on the United States National Register of Historic Places for architectural significance. Henry's son, Jerry, has since taken over for his dear father.

For Mike (ten), Bob (nine), and me the days would often be painfully long. With Mom out of town working the majority of the day at the Warm Springs State Mental Hospital, and no father around, we were generally forced to keep ourselves entertained, which was often a recipe for boyish trouble. Depending on the season, we could be found dodging cars as we rode sleds down snowy hills near roadways, recklessly climbing the steep Rocky Mountains—which beckoned us from either side of our house—or even "floating" the dangerously roaring Warm Springs Creek on worn, patched inner tubes we would beg local gas stations to give us.

We also found unique, if unlawful, ways to feed ourselves in typically exciting, youthful ways. What some called stealing, we simply termed "raiding gardens"! The funny thing is, back then it sounded more heroic than dastardly. Somehow, thievery didn't seem like such a crime when you were seven years old and hungry. Ironically, it was also about the only time I ever remember enjoying vegetables as a kid. These days I shudder when I think of the poor ladies and gentlemen who meticulously tended their gardens by day only to have us ravage their carrots, rhubarb, and lettuce by night. On occasion, those everaging caretakers, keeping watch by moonlight, would startle us in their watermelon patch as we helped ourselves to their delights. The voices of these garden tenders would bellow loudly as they chased us out of their produce, rakes raised above their heads. Still, it only added to the fun and excitement of our minor juvenile delinquency.

One night, however, we realized that we'd finally bitten off more than we could chew. It was the night the law was called on us. In Anaconda back in the 1960s the "law" meant Officer Dan Jancic. He was a classic, no-nonsense beat cop who delighted in tracking us juvenile offenders who'd developed a penchant for pirating produce. Like the thieves in the night we were, we'd grown carelessly bold. We'd somehow built a perfect record of cleanly escaping night after night with nothing on our hands but dirt-filled radishes and glorious stories to tell our friends later in our outdoor fortresses back home. Back then "sleeping out" meant six to eight of us huddled together, wrapped in old blankets placed on the soft and sweet deep grass of our backyard. Personally, somehow I always felt a little more secure when I was the one who got to use Dad's army-issued mummy bag to retreat into.

But on that one particular night, Officer Jancic finally found a way to arrest the neighborhood's growing garden attacks with a sneaky sortie of his own. Maybe it was the hunger, or maybe it was simply the warm, sultry late summer evening that beckoned droves of neighborhood kids to come together for one last insubordinate night of free food before the gardens became fallow for the fall and winter. Regardless, it was inevitable. Friends from all over town, from the west to the east side, commonly known as "Goosetown," gathered in customary dark clothing to pull off what was intended to be the organic heist of the summer.

As evening dawned, the gathering had become larger than life, at least in the minds of us younger than ten years old. It was a legendary following of local kids, delinquent as we were, coming together like no other night before. For Mike, Bobby, and me, it seemed like destiny. Finally, a grand opportunity for the three of us brothers to find our niche in the community.

The excitement was palpable, if brief. By creative design, luck, or simply by fluke, Officer Jancic was on to us. In fact, soon after we invaded our first garden en masse, Officer Jancic could be seen hopping the chain-link fence behind us with his gun and handcuffs glimmering in the late July moonlight. With

5

raspberry stains of guilt still fresh on our hands, Office Jancic rounded us all up with one loud, booming instruction—"Freeze everyone!"—effectively cracking the legendary fruit and vegetable case. Just like that, our uncanny pursuit of neighborhood string beans was over. We were each scolded and cursed upon that night by the long arm of the law. While no arrests were made, a quick assurance was made that we'd be handed down the worst sentence known to kids in those days: a telephone call to our parents!

Fortunately for Mike, Bobby, and me, our understanding mother was not only aware of our sinister plot from the get-go, she was also a lifelong cauliflower lover and fully complicit in the scheme! So while Mom calmly assured Officer Jancic that she would deal with her reprehensible boys in a manner she felt was most appropriate, she actually wound up dishing out our punishment by fixing us nice bowls of hot vegetable soup for the rest of the week! Mom may not have been perfect back then, but as the years went on, she became delightfully close to it. And in the most blessed way possible, she would one day find herself striving for perfection alongside the singular father figure that my brothers and I loved, admired, and needed the most.

Chapter 2:

Elders of Israel

WITH DAD STILL THOUSANDS OF MILES AWAY at war, our Anaconda apartment felt very empty that first December after settling there. Ironically, the person viewers of FOX13 TV in Salt Lake City, Utah, would one day come to know as "Happy Joe" (that was me) was anything but. During those days of insecurity and loneliness, I was often sad, scared, and quite unhappy—and so was Mom, which made things worse. Oftentimes in that old, pink apartment, in our youthful attempts to cheer her up, my brothers and I would get together and conceive a skit or comedy routine. Rudimentary as they were, the run of our minor league road shows always orchestrated laughter and good spirit. Though we were just young children, nothing made us feel happier than seeing our mother smile. While our gleeful plays provided a semblance of welcome relief, the fun run of our play, along with the laughter, was fleeting. Inevitably, the tragic reality of our situation would return to transform our comedies into tear-jerkers.

Nevertheless, while we didn't recognize fully at the time the one thing that would have helped us most—approaching the Lord as a family in prayer—we did feel His tender mercies at critical moments when we needed Him most. One such glorious present arrived gift-wrapped that first holiday season. A loving gesture from the Lord himself that would leave an infinite impact on each of us, simple as it was.

Decembers in Anaconda had a way of bringing out the bitterest of cold days, especially when the cool chill of lonesomeness had already permeated the walls of our aging apartment. While Mom's humble bank account couldn't provide much in the way of toys or candy that Christmas Eve, we did have the essentials. In this case, a small non-illuminated tree conspicuously situated on our dinner table. It was glorious in its own way and perfect for the four of us to gather around.

In the shining spirit of the season, a neighbor saw to it that Mom was given a small electronic light stand. It had a round circulating face that featured four different Christmas colors of delight—red, blue, green, and yellow. When plugged in, those plastic-coated colors, illuminated with a candescent bulb, would go 'round and 'round to effectively shine a different color on the tree with each complete rotation. It was amazingly elementary, yet within every revolution, the warm glow of hope and joy of the season filled our souls. The recognition of Christ's birth grew stronger in our hearts... even strong enough to allow us to forget those "wordly" burdens that can sometimes take our thoughts away from the true meaning of Christmas.

And so, as our old wooden wall clock struck seven, a joyous and strong spirit could be felt on that otherwise frosty night—providing the glow we needed and longed for. I could never recall us being together in church as a family, and I think it was fair to say that we knew very little of organized religion, yet it was obvious that our genuine feelings of the Lord could have come from no other source except the Holy Ghost, inspired by the Savior Himself.

> MATTHEW 7:7–8 "Ask and it shall be given you; seek and ye shall find; knock, and it shall be opened unto you."

Suddenly and wonderfully, that knock presented itself. Almost on cue as we were sitting tableside talking and laughing, a knock came on the door! I recall excitedly causing a stir by yelling something about Santa Claus, which sent our excited quartet rushing to seek an answer! The old wooden door wasn't always easy to open, even on the warmest of evenings, but we unlocked the latch and all pitched in to pull it open, and there we found two smiling young men at our door. "Hello. We're missionaries from the Church of Jesus Christ of Latter-Day Saints. Could we come in and share a message from God?"

To be perfectly honest, we may not have answered the door for these two young men any other night of the year. While religion was found in our hearts, we had never really thought of ourselves actually sitting in church. But on this night, it frankly didn't matter. Even if they had told us they were only there to fix our plumbing, *we had company on Christmas Eve, and it was awesome!*

United, we invited these elders in and sat quietly and peacefully listening to their message of love from God above. They told us of Jesus Christ's birth, and how much the Savior knew and loved each of us. With the spirit as our guide, every word rang true to us, even though it was the first time we'd ever heard it put forth in such a way. Afterwards we sang Christmas songs by the tree, and for the first time in my life, I truly felt the real joy and purpose of the season. My greatest gift that night, however, was witnessing long-absent peace and joy return to our mom. These two young men, who had unselfishly left their own lives and families for two years to bring the love of God to others, reset our lives in a way for which I will forever be thankful. Anytime you're on the Lord's errand, good things will be the result. If only Dad could have been there.

Chapter 3:

Boys of Summer

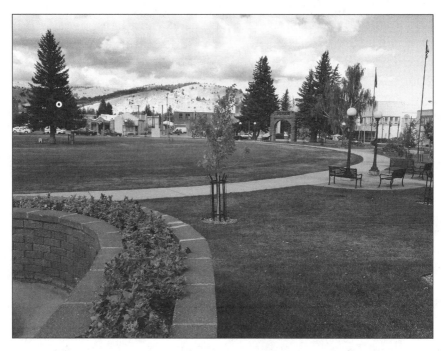

JOHN F. KENNEDY COMMONS ANACONDA, MONTANA 2017

A S THE MONTHS ROLLED ON, MANY WERE THE days I wished my dad was near, and often in ways that I'd never known of before. Early that summer, as the birds and the sunshine triumphantly returned to the Smelter City, I learned I was now old enough to sign up for Little League baseball. While I'd rarely ever played the game, I loved watching baseball games in person and on TV, and was quite mesmerized when I received my very first team uniform from the Anaconda

City League. How proud of it I was. I recall putting a few more holes in that already antiquated uniform even before the first game of the season by sporting it around the neighborhood for show. I'd wear it for pickup games, playing with friends, or even going to the Laundromat with Mom. I loved sports, and thanks to my dad's precedence, I was proud to wear a uniform. It meant I was part of a team too, and that I had a purpose.

The first team I played for was the Colts. One thing most grown-up Little Leaguers will tell you is that somehow, no matter how old we get, we can still remember virtually every player on that first team. In this case, that list included my life-long buddy Tracy Moses. I couldn't have been more proud on Opening Day, standing out in center field at John F. Kennedy Commons in the heart of Anaconda. As the national anthem played, I smacked my mitt, occasionally peeking over at Tracy in right. My only concern in the world was nervously hoping that I wouldn't drop any balls out there and let my team down. I also maintained lingering thoughts of my mother at work and my father at war—and how desperately I wished they were both there to happily cheer me on.

From as far back as I can remember, athletics played an enormous part of my life. I watched and played every game I could, often pretending to be a great athlete myself. Baseball being my first love, each spring after my first as a Little Leaguer, my heart would begin beating a little faster as I anticipated even our first practice. Through the months of long, cold winter after my first season, I even recall dreaming of a move up to Anaconda's "big leagues" (as the best athletes and town referred to it). While every young boy in town could simply sign up and be assigned to a team in the City League, the other league in town, the eight-team Jaycees League, was exclusively for the top players. To make one of those eight teams, you needed to try out and prove your ability beyond the average young man to get drafted onto a team. And though I didn't think I had a chance, I signed up for those tryouts with great enthusiasm. After all, it would be an honor for me just to be on that field. To this day I'm still not sure what Coach Steve Lane saw in me, but as good fortune would have it, he selected me to join his team back in 1969, playing for Buttrey's Foods in the coveted league.

I guess I was just about the proudest kid in town the day Coach Lane called me with the good news. While I soon found out that we weren't a good ball club at the time, it really didn't matter, because we all loved to play so much. Season after season we fought hard and had fun, but we only came away with one or two victories a year. In the infant stages of my competitive nature, after each season concluded with Buttrey's in last place, I made vows to greatly improve through devoted winter practices, alone if necessary, in my oft snow-packed backyard. Through plenty of neighborhood lawn-moving jobs, I eventually saved up a whopping five dollars to purchase a long-desired tool certain to ensure off-season success: a pitch-back machine! Since my dad never was able to play catch with me, and my brothers had no interest in baseball, I was forced to adapt my workout routine from a team aspect to an individual effort.

The pitch-back device was simply a crude metal frame that housed a 4'x4' springy net with a square in the middle. Ideally, as I pitched and hit that center square, I would be rewarded by having the ball bounced right back to me, so I devoted my efforts to getting better and better at nailing it. In time, the positive consequential effects of those efforts paid off. As I daydreamed it would hundreds of times before the next spring, that extra effort provided the very improvement and confidence I needed to help elevate my team to the Anaconda City Baseball Championship Game.

It was July 1973, and I was on a mission. After leading my team to a somewhat less-than-spectacular 5–37 season during my initial three years of Jaycees ball, I was ferociously focused on having a successful final season as a twelve-year-old. I enjoyed reasonable success batting and pitching that season, and more important, I was blessed with some fine teammates. Our team's biggest claim to fame was Jim "Jimmer" Estes. Jimmer was an awesome shortstop and a pretty fine pitcher as well.

Plus he had the pedigree. Jim was my neighbor on Ogden Street in what was called Anaconda's "new addition." Much more important, Jim was the nephew of the late, great Wayne Estes. Wayne was a legendary Anaconda hero, and the 6'6" basketball forward went on to become an All-American star at Utah State University from 1963 to 1965. By the time his collegiate career ended, Estes finished as one of the Aggies' all-time leading scorers and rebounders. Along with being recognized as one of the nation's top players, Wayne was also projected to be an NBA first-round draft pick, most likely to be drafted by the Los Angeles Lakers. Under the scenario, Wayne would have wound up a teammate alongside such famous NBA players as Wilt Chamberlain, Jerry West, and Gail Goodrich on the Lakers future NBA championship teams. But that scenario was not to be, because of a dreadfully tragic accident one night following his greatest game at USU.

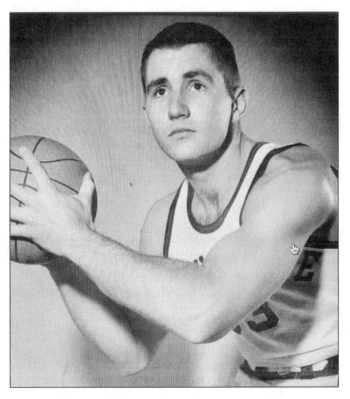

Former Utah State All-American Wayne Estes

13

During his last game ever, against the University of Denver in the old Nelson Field House, Wayne reached the 2,000-point mark of his illustrious career by scoring a whopping forty-eight points. However, after the game, Wayne and some friends stopped at the scene of a car accident near campus. While crossing the street, Wayne inadvertently brushed his head against a downed power line and was fatally electrocuted. No one alive in Anaconda then would ever fully get over the hometown hero's painful and untimely death. His gym shoes and shorts were proudly on display at the Marcus Dally Hotel in the town's city center for years to come. I often dropped by that shrine to Wayne by myself just to read and reread the many newspaper clippings in that glass case.

To this day, fans in Logan, Utah—the home of USU—also fondly remember Wayne as one of the greatest athletes ever to wear a Utah State University uniform. In May 2013 USU announced the construction of the $9.7 million Wayne Estes Center on the USU campus, which now serves as the practice facility for the Aggies men's and women's basketball teams. Silently, I played that year for Jimmy and the memory of Wayne.

Rounding out our Buttrey's baseball team was "Jumpin'" Joe Wolpert on third, Mike "Pickett" Gransberry behind the plate, Kerry Hatcher over on first, and Henry Lussey's boy, Jerry, out in center. That combination of blossoming talent and excited young men turned out to be enough to turn our one-time group of Bad News Bears into a suddenly respected and occasionally even feared baseball team. While we lost our share of games that season, something was different about our confidence and determination for the games. By the middle of the season, after finally ditching our "never-can-win" mind-set, things changed almost quicker than we could believe. Along with winning games, we began feeling like champions! Possible delusions of grandeur, since we still had one of the worst records in town, but in our minds we believed we were much better than we had been.

In fact, for the first time ever, Game 1 of the postseason city tournament wasn't something we dreaded but something we eagerly and confidently looked forward to. Oh, how

I remember the fire in my belly as the game approached. All that time tossing worn-out baseballs to my now-worn-out pitch-back machine in snowy, twenty-five-degree weather had paid off. Coach Lane even saw fit to select me as his starting pitcher in Game 1, and it turned out to be the greatest game of my life.

Some of the best athletes in town played for our opponent, mighty First Security Bank, but for some reason I wasn't concerned. Oh, sure, we'd never beaten the bank in my four years in the league, and yes, almost every game against them saw us routinely dismissed via the mercy 10-run rule, but this one was different. Pitch after pitch, batter after batter, I grew more and more confident. Even in the bottom of the last inning, I continued throwing hard and right at the center square of my catcher's target. When the final strikeout occurred, our entire team stormed the mound in great joy and excitement. It was as though we'd won the World Series. Equally priceless was the look on our parents' faces that we'd put our minds to something and pulled it off. While I sadly wished my mom didn't have to work that night, I was proud of her for doing what was needed to keep our family afloat.

A day later, I fondly remember sitting on my front porch in the glow of a particularly warm sunlight. There I read, over and over, the *Anaconda Leader*'s report of that great big Little League upset.

Imagine, I thought, just one more win and I would be pitching in the spot I'd always dreamed of: the championship game! Surely winning the championship would make me the happiest boy in town.

Well, we got that critical second win just one night later, upsetting the Job Corps team that had also destroyed us twice during the regular season. The wildest dream of my childhood was going to come true when Coach Lane told the team after that semifinals upset that I was going to be the starting pitcher in the title game!

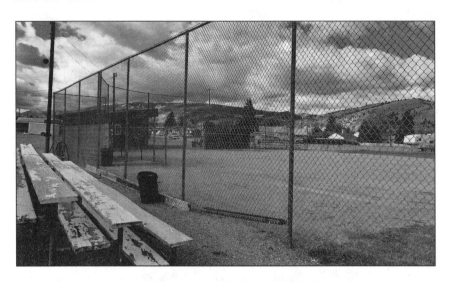

JAYCEE BASEBALL FIELD (Now known as MARTY MAY FIELD)
ANACONDA, MONTANA 2017

With a whole week to wait until the championship series, I spent hours receiving congratulations from friends and neighbors. My tiny dose of fame had not only resulted in tremendous personal achievements, small as they were, but had also given me my first opportunity to battle pride.

The more I thought of the game, the more I began to feel the weight of my growing ego. Small butterflies began feeling more like small birds in my stomach each night as I anticipated the big game. Those extra days only served to offer extra time for anxieties to build, which led to sleepless nights. While I was as thrilled and excited as I'd ever been, I was also more nervous than ever. Each minute of the day and night I would go over in my mind ways to walk to the mound, methods of making my windup "cooler," and even what I would wear under my uniform. The way I saw it, the shirt under my jersey was always critical to me, a stubbornly superstitious ballplayer. Unfortunately, because it was the hideous early '70s, I went with my wildly colored, semi-psychedelic long-sleeve shirt that had been with me for every regular-season game we had won. It was, after all, my lucky shirt that had seen us through wins on two occasions when it was actually snowing! It was nice, warm, and cozy then, but it was highly inappropriate for the eighty-degree conditions the night of the finals.

Finally, the big day arrived. It was far and away the best-attended game of the season. I arrived a couple hours early to get the most out of living my dream—even though minute by minute it became nightmarish, considering how increasingly I was allowing myself to be filled with fear and anxiety.

Our opponent, First National Bank, was loaded with the coolest kids in town. Their star was a guy my age who I'd never even met but who I knew of: Tommy "Obe" Oberweiser, who was idolized by everyone. His father was a great high school football coach, and Obe had older brothers who were also sports stars. Only eight months prior, we were opposing quarterbacks in the city Grade School Football Championship Game. That was supposed to be my great chance to show him and the rest of our town how cool I was. Tom's St. Paul team had defeated every opponent that year and generally were considered to have the best talent in town. Try as I might that late afternoon on the Mitchell Stadium gridiron, I let my Dwyer team down in a 12–8 loss I would never get over. But now I had a second chance to fully redeem all–if I could somehow bury my fears.

Decades later, yet with the game still fresh in his memory, Obe recalled to me something special about that game that surprised me. He said, "Our coach, Joe Mennicucci, was very aware that you were their best player. When he learned that you would be pitching, he actually turned to me and said, 'We're going to pitch you against Buttrey's. I want it to be our best against their best.' I'll never forget him saying that because it made me proud and very nervous at the same time." If only I had known that even my boyhood hero at the time was feeling almost exactly the way I was.

To me it was as glorious a sight as I could imagine. There on the pitcher's mound that night, I soaked it all in. After all, to me the moment meant much more than just a game. The bleachers were packed so full that many of the hundreds of fans showing up needed to drive and park their cars all around the outside of the fences to get a good seat as the players took the field to observe the national anthem. This one game appeared to

17

have drawn just about everyone in town—including my mom! I believe, since it was on a Saturday night, it was one of the first games she was able to attend, and I was proud as I could be looking out and seeing her glowingly looking back at me. If only the game could have ended right there.

Looking back at it over the years, I somehow found myself embroiled in many spotlight opportunities, but in very few of them did I ever feel like I was fully worthy of being there. Too often such distrust in myself morphed into anxiety, leading me to some type of self-fulfilling failure. Such was the case in this final game of my Little League career. After all the pomp and circumstance afforded the two teams that qualified for this final night of play, I now had to approach the pitching mound and not only prove that I could lead my team to a win but that I could even step up onto that hill without feeling like I was going to lose my lunch.

All I can say about my first few pitches is that I probably couldn't have thrown the ball into the ocean if you'd spotted me the beach. I'd spent so much time that previous week imagining how incredible it would be to be there that when the critical moment finally arrived, it was more of an out-of-body experience than reality. I've heard it said that life can be 99 percent expectation and just 1 percent realization. Such was the case for me that warm evening as both the stars and the dark clouds came out in Anaconda.

I began a string of wild pitches so crazy that not even the hot dog vendor could take his eye off me for fear of even himself being beaned. Not only did I walk the very first batter, none of those four pitches were even remotely near the strike zone. While the next batter played the odds and swung at a wild pitch I'd tossed, eventually he recognized the law of averages and patiently awaited his own free ride to first.

Coach Lane, more Ward Clever than Sparky Anderson, called for a timeout, and as tranquilly as he knew how, he approached the mound to calm me down. "Joe," he counseled, "I know you're a fine pitcher and you know it too. So I want you to go back on that mound and throw hard like you've been doing all season and let the chips fall where they may."

I trusted him, and I knew I *could* do it too. I just didn't think there was a chance that I *would*. Nevertheless, I got back onto that Little League hill and stared down the next batter with great intensity. After taking peeks at the two runners impatiently waiting to advance, even yelling to me to throw another ball over the catcher's head, I angrily began the most intimidating windup I knew. The whole time reminding myself, "Pitch this one as hard as you can!" Which I did—only to see my fastball wrongly break into the batter's right leg. After jumping around a bit in pain, he took off to first amidst some slight boos directed at me as I watched every base fill with still no outs on the scoreboard. It truly became not only the worst spot I'd ever been in as a baseball pitcher but also one of the worst moments of my young life. My heart broke knowing that any pitch from that point could give First National Bank the lead.

The crowd cheered and jeered as I then went on to walk batter after batter. The mental torture was severe. I hated letting people down, let alone myself. Inside I was begging the coach to come end this misery.

Somewhere around the fourth inning, with our team being humbled by several runs, I approached the plate as a batter. A quick glance over to Mom just before stepping into the batter's box provided just what I needed: a warm smile and look from her that gave me great confidence. I knew I was going to get a hit! Standing there, despite all that had happened that night, my fears took a hike. I recall swinging as hard as I could, the results of which scorched a hard liner past second base as I joyfully wound up on first with a single. The crowd cheered, and I wondered if it would be the unlikely impetus for a dramatic rally to win!

Standing there on first base marked the first positive thing I'd done that evening since putting on my socks. Yet instead of humbly trying to be a good sport, my youthful pride urged me to begin whooping it up in a vain and unsportsmanlike attempt to distract their pitcher, Tom Oberweiser. As our next batter, "Jumpin'" Joe Wolpert, came to the plate, I had high hopes he'd blast one far enough for me to score our team's very first run. He hit the ball all right, but his connection was more of a bunt than a thundering crash. Nevertheless, I took off for

19

second with my customary reckless abandon! Some two years to the day after watching Pete Rose crash into Ray Fosse in the Major League Baseball All-Star Game, I was prepared to recreate history and change the course of the game with my hardball base-running skills. Despite the fact that their second baseman already had been thrown the ball for the force out, I intended to force my will by crashing over the top of him with every intent of jarring the ball loose.

If that sounds terribly unsportsmanlike, it's because it was. As the umpire inevitably called me out, I'd had it. The bottled-up frustrations and defeats of my entire life suddenly spilled out uncontrollably onto that dirt field. Instead of peacefully walking away, I began taking out my rage on the guy who tagged me out, and soon a near-bench-clearing brawl ensued on the very scene I'd intended to be my finest hour. Obe joined in but only to correctly try and maintain peace and order. While I was prepared and eager to throw a punch at the one player in the league who I'd always idolized, he was merely trying to do the right thing. What was supposed to be one of the greatest nights of my life quickly turned into one of my worst embarrassments and failures.

There was a time that night, in a moment I had dreamt of 1,000 times before, that I felt I had everything I thought was needed to be happy in life. But painfully the lesson I learned was that it's not enough to simply desire a situation to happen—I needed to become the type of person who could do all he could to rise to challenges, and then humbly accept the Lord's will.

In hindsight, I can see that I did win at least one positively memorable thing that night. Despite the inauspicious start to our friendship, even to this day Obe and I very fondly look back at the moments of that night. The scars of those precious lessons, though painfully earned, now provide a healing balm as we slide into our older years. Our laughing and reminiscing have now replaced Bengay as our go-to method of feeling good and overcoming pain—the kind of stuff that great, lifelong friendships are made of. We now fully recognize these blessings.

Not surprisingly, many decades later, in what would become the single-most-nightmarish moment of my life, Obe would again show up to help maintain peace and order.

Chapter 4:

Wayne and Lamar

O NE DAY BACK IN LATE 1972, AS I SAT ALONE AT
home watching television, the Lord told me, "You are
never alone."

Seemingly content to waste my days away in listless leisure,
I was suddenly caught off guard by the shadow of two person-
ages approaching my door through the veil of the front window.
This stirred me to sit up and curiously take note as multiple
knocks came on the door. "Knock and it shall be opened to
you" was one of the few scriptures I recalled at the time. I was
convinced it was either a couple of my friends or an acquain-
tance of my mom there to drop something off. As I opened it I
found it to be both, and that initial shock of seeing who it was
is still quite vivid to me these many years later.

There on the doorstep stood a kindly gentleman of around
forty years old next to a younger boy who was my age. I
knew he was my age because I knew him. Boy, did I. Lamar
Nelson was his name. While I'm not sure if we'd ever really
talked to each other before as friends, Lamar and I had
attended elementary school together ever since I'd enrolled
at W.K. Dwyer Elementary back in '69. Lamar and I were
different people. Not Tracy Moses and I different; more like
night-and-day different. While I spent most of the school day
honing my skills of delinquent humor to impress classmates
by disrupting class and leading chaos on the playground,
Lamar was essentially my extreme opposite, bless his heart.
Not only was Lamar an extremely well-behaved young man
who could generally be seen with a smile on his face and a
schoolbook in his hands; he went about his day sporting a

gentle and patient personality that went hand in hand with that full-time grin on his face. "What is *he* smiling about?" I often though to myself.

Though he was big, rotund, and physically strong, the trait that bewildered me was the loving, calm, and peaceful way Lamar carried himself all day at school. While I was prideful and mindful only of myself, Lamar seemed oblivious to the need of seeking public opinion to validate himself.

I loved and respected that in him but never really envisioned a day when I would come to be so at peace with myself. While I hadn't previously realized it, Lamar likely developed such honorable characteristics through his own trials and challenges in life. He was no stranger to displaying patience and dignity several times a day, and in a most heroic fashion.

You see, Lamar had a younger brother, Wayne, who was mentally challenged—although that's not the politically incorrect term many of the schoolyard bullies used to refer to him back then. Thankfully, we've come a long way as a society in how we treat beautiful but challenged children such as Wayne. Nevertheless, too many of his classmates in that day and age spent their wistful minutes of recess seeking cruel ways to cover their own insecurities by unkindly making a mockery of Wayne's talk and walk.

As intent on gaining public favor and laughter as I was, I still shied away from joining a crowd so eager to belittle. Casting insults in such a situation was not for me. Besides, I'd privately developed a quiet respect watching those two brothers deal with their troubling times. However, I was guilty of not ever stepping up to these rowdy boys and insisting they put a stop to the endless tormenting of Wayne. I guess I was, shamefully, just too afraid of either ruining my limited stature with them or perhaps receiving a bloody nose.

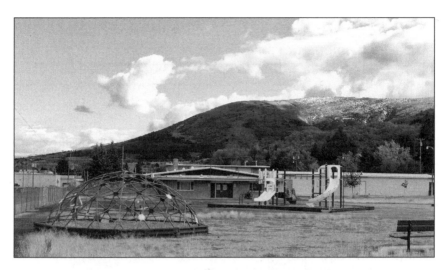

W.K. DWYER ELEMENTARY. ANACONDA, MONTANA

Thankfully, there was one who admirably stood by Wayne's side day after day, in a way that always warmed my heart. I secretly marveled at the love and dignity Lamar personified as he put on the armor of being "his brother's keeper." Somber yet stately, Lamar would valiantly endure the tempest of some of the ugliest storms of name-calling and mockery one could imagine. Almost daily, a few or more of the school "tough guys" would surround Wayne to openly mock his limited mental condition. Oftentimes many of our classmates would gather to join in and laugh openly, or perhaps cry a bit in their hearts at the sadness of it all. Either way, I'm confident that I wasn't the only one who would cheer inside at the eventual sight of brother Lamar, with a sincere smile and large heart, tenderly walking past the oppressors to put his arm around Wayne and escort him away from the hurtful talk and insulting laughter.

"Hello, Joe, we're from the Church of Jesus Christ of Latter-Day Saints," the gentleman at the door said. "My name is Ed Holloran; I'm a young men's leader. You probably know Lamar?"

Yes, *that* Lamar.

"Lamar has just been set apart as president of the Aaronic Priesthood Quorum in the local ward of the Church of Jesus Christ of Latter-Day Saints and immediately asked if you would consider being his first counselor."

23

I didn't have the slightest idea what they were talking about, and for a moment, I even considered slamming the door and hiding. But then, for whatever reason, I heard myself say, "Yes, I will"… and I did. I shook hands with them and felt a strong glow in me that I'd rarely ever felt before. This would do absolutely nothing for me as far as school popularity, but strangely, it did everything for me as far as providing tranquility and inner peace. A few months later, I would receive the Aaronic Priesthood as well, the way all others do who are commissioned of God, through direct laying on of hands by one already ordained with the proper authority. It was a very happy day for me—even though I still didn't discuss it much with my mother or brothers. I had become somewhat independent by then, and at the time, religion wasn't something we openly discussed.

Chapter 5:

Friends for Life

As TIME ROLLED ON, MY LOVE OF THE LORD continued to grow—as did my recognition that I needed Him. That inner desire drove me on a search to find Him and His Spirit wherever I thought I could, which included the attendance of as many religious services as I could find, possibly in an effort to relive that Christmas Eve in our apartment. From Catholic Mass to Baptist meetings, I took it all in—and developed a love for those parishioners who attended. Often I would intently watch their faces in worship, many so often gripped in anguish, need, and desire for blessings that they kneeled in abject humbleness to directly commune with the Lord Almighty. During those years I saw firsthand how they truly recognized a need to seek a togetherness with the Lord in whatever ways they felt they knew how.

Mike Strizich and Dan Roche were two of my good friends back in the early 1970s. Probably the two coolest kids in town, so no real surprise that I sought them out as constant companions. I enjoyed the fact that they could be cool *and* attend their church. I recall many Sundays spent with them attending church services that their families were dedicated to. Plus it was handy. At the time, the Catholic St. Paul's Church held mass immediately behind our new home on 1616 Ogden Ave. Dan's mom and dad, Juanita and John, were strong members of the community and always showed me true Christian love and warmth. They also showed me how important it is for a family to be together. I was encouraged and delighted to attend Catholic Mass. At the time, their services were held in a Lutheran Church building while a new Holy Family Church was being built.

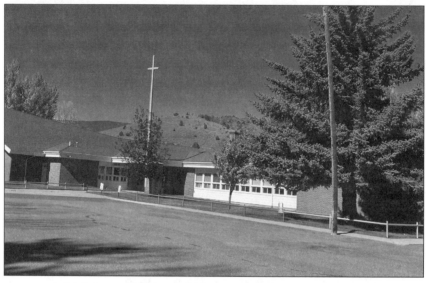

HOPE LUTHERAN CHURCH, ANACONDA, MONTANA

To this day I can still close my eyes and see and listen to that congregation. I even recall songs sung there those forty years ago—and the deep devotion those good, God-fearing people had. Two of the parishioners, Howie Thompson and Don Loranger, became favorites of mine through their music. The duo kept a sweet spirit flowing with cherubic voices that were deep and strong; it made me want to be a better person just by listening and feeling that happiness. I still sing one of their songs, "Lord Help Me Jesus," to myself from time to time. I was a bit of a wild child by then but always kept my feelings for the Lord close by.

We all seemed to grow up fast in Anaconda. I was given a taste of how fast things moved while attending the opening night of the high school football season in 1973. As our local Anaconda Copperheads team kicked off the year, some of my classmates chose to kick off a new series of questionable activities—certainly for children that age. Even though I was only in the seventh grade, some of my peers asked me to chip in that night for a keg of beer. The plan was to meet postgame at a previously agreed-upon location on the secluded mountainside behind the stadium. At the time, I didn't even know what a keg was, and even though I had plenty of anxiety over drinking at my age, I chipped in my two dollars just to be a part of the gang. Drinking alcohol during that era, and in that town, was actually somewhat accepted—even expected. Given I had been on a lifelong search for acceptance—and some semblance of happiness and peace—maybe this would provide it?

Dan Roche was a classic Anaconda kid who had some character traits that I gravitated toward as an early teen. He was a tough, good-looking guy's guy who also had an exciting way with the girls who eagerly chased after him—boy, did he know how to talk to them! We met in seventh grade and were fairly inseparable for the next two to three years. Dan shared my penchant for boyish mischief. The youngest son of an Anaconda police officer, Danny had the ability to pull off some of our wildest times with just a sly grin and his charming personality. To this day, I love Dan, but we both recognize that living close to the Lord provides more joy and peace than rowdy days skipping school and chasing gals. As life wore on, we both learned painful lessons from poor decisions made during those young days.

Mike was also a strong influence on me during those teen years. Pound for pound the bravest and toughest kid I ever knew. He was bold in his speech and able to back it up with a left or a right if needed! Along with that strength, he carried great charm. Those two qualities, combined with his overwhelming talent as an athlete, made him one of the greatest and most successful men ever to leave Anaconda. To this day, I stay in close contact with Mike, sometimes sharing our previous "boys will be boys" moments from our childhood days in Anaconda with a laugh and a smile. Striz was his nickname then, and it still is, but it may easily have been Winner.

Mike secured traits early in his life that I always appreciated. Many of those he credits to his strong mother and father. They never allowed him to lazily waste the day away; instead they saw to it that Mike worked hard and often. Each day of the week, even very early before school, Mike would be up delivering newspapers by 4:00 AM. I marveled at such dedication and discipline and stayed close to him, hoping one day I could grasp his secret—a secret that would ultimately allow him to become a very wealthy and successful man. Striz's secret, as it turned out, had nothing to do with athletics or boyish charm; it was simply good old-fashioned education and hard work.

Ultimately, his dedication to learning and achieving would not only supply him with all the money he could ever dream of, but it also supplied him the ability to jump into his very own private jet one day on September 2, 2016. It was a hurried and emotional flight that saw him land in Ogden, Utah, before an equally hurried drive to the emergency room of McKay Dee Hospital. There he would rush to my hospital bedside after he being shockingly informed only hours earlier by family members that I may not live through the day.

Chapter 6:

Domestic Disturbance

A S I BECAME A TEENAGER, THE CHALLENGES OF life seemed to compound. The harder I pushed along, the more I felt opposition to my progress. Fright and anxiety were too often my closest companions. I never did get over the feeling of being alone after my parents divorced. Mom was a sharp, wonderful lady with much to offer; she eventually did remarry, if only to have some semblance of a father figure around the house and someone to help with expenses.

But as many seeking marriage under such circumstances likely find out, true love and devotion from a partner are most important and necessary; otherwise, the relationship is not going to last. We all found that out sometime after Mom married again. Following the initial positive courtship, her new husband turned out to be a heavy drinker and abusive, which added a very unwelcome set of problematic issues and created even more depression for each of us.

Adding to my heartaches of that day were the many nights of unrest. Many weekends, instead of going out socializing with all my friends, I instead felt a chilling obligation to stay close to home and do what I could to make sure Mom was safe. Most nights I would even sleep by the door of my bedroom, listening until early in the morning occasionally to make sure the arguments he would start didn't spill into his physical violence, which all too often they did. In that case, I would either sit paralyzed in fright and guilt, or possibly run out through the living room to phone the police for help. Sadly, in those days the police would simply come to the door and ask the husband to tone it down a little, after which the abuse could often continue even worse.

Finally, one day as my brothers Mike and Bob were with me downstairs watching television, we heard the awful sound of violence upstairs. It was clear what was happening again. But this time we decided enough was enough. While we stood by the door for a moment listening to what was transpiring, we recognized that if something wasn't done immediately, Mom's life, and that of the child she was then carrying, would be in jeopardy. We had garnered enough evidence to take matters into our own youthful hands, and finally we added to that a sense of steely determination. Whether it was the angst and anxiety of the moment, or just an inkling of the courage our father used when he went into battle in precarious situations, the three of us burst through the door and onto a frightening scene of physical and emotional battery. Mike, three years older than me but still a young teenager, courageously moved forward to protect Mom with fists flying. Plenty of pent-up anger would be released as punishment was delivered. While I was convinced it was a noble and needed effort on our part, I'd previously felt such an effort would be unwinnable considering the opposition we were going up against. However, Mike and Bob were determined, and eventually took the abuser to the ground and humbled him. He apologized and recognized he'd been defeated.

Shortly after that, Mom realized that as much as she hated ending another marriage, she had absolutely no choice here. After this divorce, we were all happier—but back to being alone. Mom still worked, leaving us boys on our own most days. I found many ways to occupy my time, but not all those things were positive—and most would lead me to increased anxiety and unhappiness.

In time, however, in His infinite wisdom and love, the Lord would provide the only perfect man for Mom to return into her life, and ours.

Chapter 7:

BYU QB Gifford Nielson

A S THE YEARS ROLLED ON, I HELD TO MY WORD to work beside Lamar in church. Though I received a considerable amount of consternation from my friends for doing so, I "held to the iron rod" as best I could, often forgoing high school parties and various other temptations to keep myself from mischief. I didn't like to drink alcohol or have my mind altered in ways that I knew were wrong. I also had too much respect for the young women who I was around, and grew to fear any thoughts that might lead me to be disrespectful to them.

Despite the occasional negative reactions from friends and acquaintances at school, I loved feeling peace, joy, and happiness in church attendance, even though I hadn't ever fully read either the Bible or *The Book of Mormon*.

One Sunday a month, the ward would hold a fast and testimony meeting in which members of the congregation would voluntarily give up food and water for a twenty-four-hour period and use the money they saved to help feed the needy. After their lengthy fast, the congregation would feel sufficiently humbled and ultimately more appreciative and worthy of the Lord's Holy Spirit. Then, in the church meeting, the members would have an opportunity to stand before others and bear the feelings of their soul publicly to help others feel of that love. Sacrifices have long been a successful way for man to show his love, trust, and faith in God. When fast and testimony meetings would occur, though I rarely fasted myself, I often marveled at those strong people who stood before others in the chapel to proclaim, "I have a testimony that God and Jesus

Christ live, and that this is true!" I thought to myself, *I wish I could have a testimony!*

One day, I finally got up enough courage to ask a young woman in the ward, Lori Smith, to tell me how I could attain such a great gift. Lori was a sweet and kind young lady who often spoke of her testimony as she helped others. I knew her mother and father as very fine people who were very positive toward me in all ways, so I guess I felt comfortable asking her such a personal question. Her response was, "One good way to get a testimony is to go up and bear it before others; in other words, try to put into words what and how you are feeling." That sounded nice and appropriate, but in my ignorance, I still didn't think I had the slightest idea what to say—or even what a testimony was. The Lord clearly knew that, and in His method of "line upon line" and "precept upon precept," I was blessed greatly when a wonderful new family moved into the ward about that very time. To say they became instrumental to my life and search for the knowledge I was so eager to receive would truly be an understatement.

George and Delores Miller were two of the finest people I'd ever known. They were also members of this church. They were the parents of six fine children. I marveled at, and now confess small jealousies over, the way they would all gather together for a family meal each night at dinnertime and share a sincere prayer seeking grace. It was classic! George had the full love and respect of his family; he was a strong leader whose advice I often sought, even though it was also clear that his wonderful wife, Delores, was every bit the true family leader he was!

Among the memorable children in the Miller home was oldest son Doug, who turned out to be the perfect friend for me at the time. He knew the gospel and did his best to live it—but still had enough minor mischief in him to allow me to transition smoothly into the young man I wanted to be. He was a year older than me, but we were quite the same in most other aspects. As a junior at Anaconda High, he once invited me to spend a weekend with him at the school formerly known as Ricks College in Idaho. There he was going to take a written quiz to submit to the church prior to receiving a mission call.

Again, I had no idea what that meant, but he spiced things up by informing me that his older sister had set up dates for us in Rexburg, and the opportunity to date a college gal at my age was rather attractive. During the four-hour drive there, we spoke plenty of what a mission was, but the way back was mostly focused on how I tipped over my soda on my date when reaching for french fries. After that we couldn't get out of that town quicker. Doug's younger sister, Andrea, was also a perfect example to me. She made it clear that a young woman of God was to hold herself with great dignity and purpose, and was to respect herself in all ways. I was then, and remain today, fully impressed and in awe of those high standards she held on to, and still does. I never felt worthy to ask such a model young woman to date, or even to hold hands, but I've never forgotten those strong values she tightly held on to, and I eventually would proudly encourage such traits in my daughters.

Not long after our weekend at Ricks College, while attending a sacrament meeting at the Anaconda ward one evening in the late 1970s (just prior to the church going to the "block system" of Sunday meetings), I overheard a fortuitous discussion by two members of the congregation in the foyer. One spoke of an amazing college quarterback who had thrown six touchdown passes *in one game* the day before! Being a tremendous sports fan, and one who had high hopes of being a TV sportscaster one day, I immediately came over to join in on the discussion. "Six touchdown passes in one game?" I asked. "Who, where, when?" In those days, the old running game philosophy of three yards and a cloud of dust ruled offenses in college and professional games. I was informed that the quarterback who had pulled off that prolific passing game was a guy named Gifford Nielson, who played for Brigham Young University." I said, "BYU? What's that?"

Gifford Nielson went on to be named a college football All-American at BYU before turning professional and playing for the NFL Houston Oilers. Statistically, he held many of the highest-regarded college football records in the nation, and ushered in a long line of All-American QBs at BYU. That list includes former NFL stars Marc Wilson, Jim McMahon, Steve Young, Robbie Bosco, and Heisman Trophy winner Ty Detmer.

33

Nearly thirty years after that conversation in the ward foyer, I would meet Gifford at the Provo MTC as we were both tearfully dropping off our sons for LDS missions. We shook hands and talked during one of the more challenging days of our lives to that point. Seeing your own son leave for two full years to help bless the lives of others can be a difficult moment.

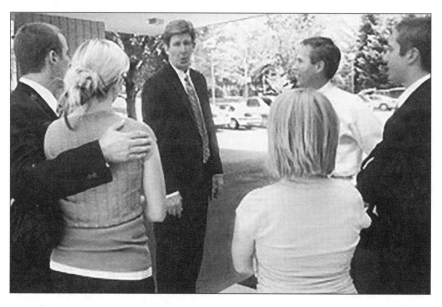

Former BYU and NFL Q.B. Gifford Nielsen meeting with Matt, Michelle, Randee, Tyler and myself outside the Provo MTC.
(Nancy taking the picture)

The great Gifford Nielson is now a general authority in the Church of Jesus Christ of Latter-Day Saints.

Chapter 8:

Living with Dad

TOWARD THE END OF MY SOPHOMORE YEAR OF high school in Anaconda, increasing thoughts of my tortured dad being without the opportunity of having any of his sons growing up by his side began to haunt me. In just two years I would be graduating, with none of us boys ever having known the joys of being together during our school days as father and son. Even more important, I was concerned about his well-being. While I was finally making headway in my efforts to survive my teenage years, he continued to battle serious depression issues inflicted by fresh memories of war. From what little I knew of his negative lifestyle, I felt his very life could be in jeopardy.

Growing up it was very easy for me to blame and even despise him occasionally for not caring enough to be there for me when I truly needed a father. At the time, I simply didn't know any better than to feel anger toward him, or even a sense that I was betrayed. He was never around for Christmas, ball games, or any of my birthdays, and rarely did he phone or visit. What kind of a father would behave like that? Was I even loved or thought of?

Granted, I was impressed when I heard of him living through nightmarish episodes of being shot down in helicopters on three different occasions during the war. He'd been a passenger in choppers that were attempting to transport him to various harrowing Special Forces missions near the North Vietnamese border. But to me, those were merely neat and heroic acts that routinely made up the life of soldiers, like the thrilling and patriotic war movies I'd seen at the theater. Seemingly nothing but excitement and glory filled his days, while I faced daily problems alone at home. Essentially, while he was out there leading a breathtaking life, I was home suffering in ways he didn't take time to consider or care about.

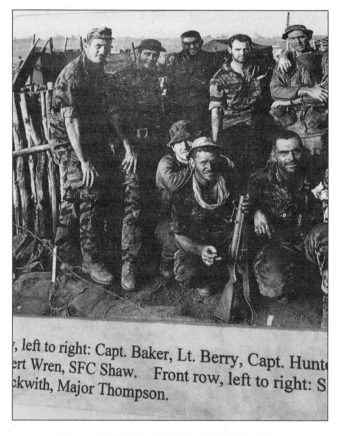

, left to right: Capt. Baker, Lt. Berry, Capt. Hunt
rt Wren, SFC Shaw.   Front row, left to right: S
ckwith, Major Thompson.

WAR PICTURE OF DAD IN VIETNAM
Robert Wren pictured with fellow U.S. Special Forces Green
Beret members at Plei Mei ~ site of the first major confrontation
between our soldiers and the communist North Vietnamese Army.

One of Dad's "exciting" episodes occurred back in April 1966. But as I would later learn, excitement and glory were far from his mind at the time.

Dad was part of the U.S. Army's very first Delta Project. That was a U.S. fighting group so exclusive that only a few in a hundred men who attempted to qualify would actually receive the honor of being one of the nation's first-ever Special Forces

Green Berets. Many brave men attempted to meet the Green Beret standard, but only a small percentage ever did. The U.S. Army decided it needed an ultra-elite force for most of its most harrowing missions.

Dad was on a dark and somber mission over a steamy jungle that overflowed with enemy soldiers that spring day in 1966. An army H-34 helicopter was carrying two pilots, a crew chief, and two door gunners, as well as a well-trained six-man fighting team that included my dad. They were courageously flying one of many high-risk missions over enemy territory. Suddenly, in the middle of a furious enemy gunfire assault at just 500 feet above the ground, the copilot took a bullet to his chest. From there, attempts to safely land the chopper were futile.

As the H-34 rapidly lost altitude and essentially began falling from the sky, Dad and the other soldiers were violently tossed about inside in a scene no action movie could ever recreate. The pilot attempted to abort, but intense enemy machine gun fire sent the aircraft tumbling hopelessly out of control toward the ground, grinding through tree branches as the engine was losing full power. Dad later recalled high-pitched chopper blade sounds as they eerily churned into the deep elephant grass covering the ground. As the grinding sound of twisted metal and blades finally came to a stop, the realization of their ghastly predicament had only just begun.

Most of the men on board, at least those who survived, could neither move nor walk—having suffered injuries too gruesome to imagine. One of the door gunners could be heard moaning loudly, his right thighbone protruding from his skin.

Prior to leaving on each of these potentially deadly assignments, Dad was always outfitted with a small .25 caliber automatic handgun. It was designed to rapidly shoot four bullets in a row. The weapon, in reality, had two possible purposes. He could either use it to defend himself in the event that he felt he had a chance to survive against the enemy that day, or he was to use it on himself if need be. Being killed, as awful as that could be, took second in line of concern for a Green Beret. His most important goal was to make sure the enemy wouldn't be able to capture him alive for interrogation. Most of the men involved in that mission died there by morning.

Later in my life, as Dad felt I was old enough to handle it, he would relay several other horrific stories of his enemy encounters. Those experiences were both shocking and humbling to me as I recognized that the repercussions of unforgettable horrible experiences like that were actually the reason I grew up without a father. Decorations of heroism at war abounded, as Dad was an absolute hero in every sense, many times unselfishly saving the lives of those valiant men he fought beside. Ultimately he became one of the most decorated soldiers of all time from the state of Montana—earning two Purple Hearts, the Distinguished Service Award, the Bronze Star, and various other recognitions for heroism and valor. In 2015 a ground stone with his name and multiple honors on it was embedded at a new Vietnam memorial park constructed in Hamilton, Montana, where he grew up.

Chapter 9:

Nancy

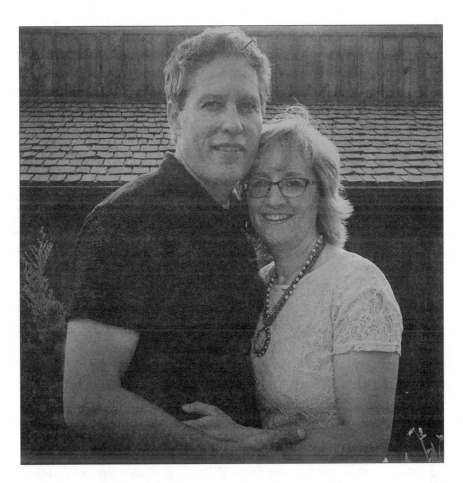

Nancy, my beautiful wife of 38 years and counting.

I'd never really thought of myself as much of a romantic growing up, but how else would you describe my love of my wife, Nancy?

Nancy Moodry was her maiden name—a name synonymous with success in Anaconda. Her father, Fred Moodry, was an icon there in Anaconda. As a devoted teacher, football and wrestling coach, and ultimately the superintendent of schools at the young age of forty-three, he became legendary in his own time. Nancy was the prettiest and most popular girl in her class. She had four brothers and two sisters, each of whom was well-known and well-thought-of in town.

As a freshman in high school, I achieved a great athletic goal when I made the varsity AHS wrestling team. It was one of the proudest days of my life to that point. I can easily remember the emotions and stresses that filled my mind during my first tournament. It was held at Butte High School, and I was very scared as I sat on the bench awaiting my match. But one thing that took my mind off my own worries was a booming voice from way up in the crowd. Two of Nancy's brothers, Mike and Tom, were each on the varsity team with me that season in 1976. They were older, more experienced, and had a father who attended every match. He was a big, strong man who friends and family referred to as the town's best friend, who was more of a teddy bear. But his voice shook the entire gymnasium when he would yell out words of advice and encouragement to his two boys from the stands. I loved it and secretly pretended he was my dad too, using those great words of wisdom as they pertained to my match. It gave me confidence, and I actually went out and won my very first match.

Just two weeks later, Fred would suffer a massive heart attack in the very school that would one day be named after him. Within an hour he would be pronounced dead at the tender age of forty-four.

As a testament to the love they had for him, virtually the entire grieving town of Anaconda turned out for the funeral. So large was the mourning crowd that they had to hold the funeral inside the AHS Memorial Gymnasium for sufficient seating. Immediately after the services, as I was walking toward home alone, I stopped and watched silently as the car carrying

Fred's wife and seven children drove past me up to Sunnyside Mortuary Cemetery. As I looked inside the windows, I found heavy sadness in all of their eyes. My heart ached for them.

Three years later, after having returned to Anaconda after living with my dad during my junior year, I was back at Memorial Gym. I had intentionally kept a low profile at school those first several months back, hoping to stay out of any type of trouble. Still, I was competitive and had a strong desire to go take a shot at trying out for the wrestling team again. I was out of shape and hadn't wrestled the past two seasons, but I strongly believed it was something that I should do. Surprisingly, after succeeding in victory during the challenge matches for varsity, I earned a spot on the first string again—and again I was able to proudly don my AHS uniform. The first tournament would be an overnight meet in Bozeman, Montana. Once again, I was very excited and very scared, but something happened that first morning as we boarded the school bus that changed my life for the better forever.

As I sat alone in the front seat on the bus, anticipating the excitement of that first match, my eye caught a young lady preparing to board our bus. Since it was a meet only for the varsity wrestlers, there was plenty of open space on board the bus for cheerleaders to ride with us—to and fortuitously Nancy Moodry, the the most adorable young woman I had ever seen (even though we'd never spoken before) was one of them. From that second on, all I could think of was her. As she came on the bus, I silently prayed—granted, against all odds—that for some reason she would choose to ignore her many other friends and sit next to me.

Always the most popular person in any crowd, Nancy walked up the stairs and glanced toward the middle of the bus. My personal prayers for her increased. She looked around again and then—wonderfully—glanced toward me. "Can I sit with you?" she asked, effectively answering my most heartfelt prayers. From that very second on, my life was never the same. In an instant I had courage, strength, and confidence. I also found purpose, joy, and happiness like I'd never known before. Later I told my mom that if I wasn't able to marry this girl, I may as well never get married at all. Fortunately, she eventually felt the same toward me. She was, and has been every minute of my life since then, the true love of my life.

My first wrestling match would provide a microcosm of the rest of our lives. While I hadn't wrestled in some thirty months, I took the great euphoria I'd felt from the warmth and sweet feelings of Nancy and turned them into a determined desire to succeed. My first match, amazingly, was going just as I'd planned. Despite being a heavy underdog to a talented opponent, I'd somehow built an early lead that surprised my coaches, teammates, and especially myself. Knowing how much I felt I needed that win to impress Nancy, I panicked a bit, and instead of staying on the offensive, I went on the defensive as the final minute of the match approached. Now very weak and tired, I simply decided to hang on for dear life and run out the clock. Surely it would be a win that would so impress this wonderful young lady that she would insist on becoming my steady date. In hindsight, those were likely not the things I should have been thinking of during my match, but there she was, alongside all the other cheerleaders just off the wrestling matt cheering away. I recall hearing every word, and thinking of how lovely she was and of all the clever and witty things I would say to her after this incredible show of strength.

Unfortunately, in the midst of all my daydreaming about my future companion, I found myself unceremoniously flipped over like a rag doll and stacked up with just seconds to go in the match.

"Pin!" shouted the official as he blew his whistle to end the match and, presumably, all of my hopes.

I was humiliated and quite certain that my dreams of an epic romance would be short-lived as I walked off being scolded by my mentor and respected head coach, Barry Huot. I didn't speak or look at Nancy at that point. How could I?

I spent the next several hours in self-pity, sadness, and disbelief at what I had foolishly and recklessly let slip away.

However, later that night, since I had lost out of the tournament and was now free to walk the streets with the others on the team who had been defeated, the Lord, in all of his mercy and love, saw to it that Nancy would come back into my life for good. In my saddest hour, walking down an empty street in

Bozeman, I heard her unmistakable voice. Nancy and the other cheerleaders were also on free time that night, heading toward a local theater to watch a movie. As my great blessing would have it, we virtually bumped into each other on the sidewalk. My shame and sorrow quickly left as Nancy enthusiastically let me know how proud she was of me for making the team and doing so well. How could it be that the Lord would love me so much as to give me this moment in time that I will always cherish and never forget? We went on to speak of many other topics that night, and even rode home together the next day on the bus, talking joyously the entire way.

I spent the following day, Sunday, thinking of her and of some way I could get back in touch with her after that glorious weekend. Suddenly it hit me. While I was now a senior who had never attended a formal high school dance in my life, the Snowball Dance prom was just a few weeks away. After conferring with some of her friends who knew her well, I learned that while Nancy had been asked to every single formal prior to that, no one had asked her to this one. I wasn't sure how she would react to an invitation from me, a nondrinking Mormon whom she had only recently met, so I employed a well-rehearsed ad-lib reconnaissance mission designed to ambush her at her place of work. Nancy was a scorekeeper for grade school basketball games, and I slyly learned of a neighbor boy whose team was scheduled to play that Monday—thus giving me the perfect alibi. That night, heart beating loudly and lovingly, I walked into the gym just as coolly and casually as I could pretend to be. Right on cue, the very first time I had the courage to glance across the gym and look at her, she was also noticing me! Even more, Nancy smiled that smile a young lady makes when they are very happy to see you, and I'm quite confident she noticed I had the same look.

During the first game break, I made my way over to her and was thrilled when she told me how happy she was to see me too. We spoke as long as we could during those timeouts, and from that point on I felt confident that I was now just a phone call away from the greatest date of my life.

Not wanting to risk her forgetting me, or having someone else ask her first, I drove straight home and began practicing

43

lines by my telephone. As I gained the courage to dial, my palms were sweating and my love-filled heart was pounding, "Hello, Nancy?" I said. "This is Joe Wren, how are you? Nancy, the Sweetheart Prom is coming up; I'd sure love to take you if you haven't been asked yet." She assured me that she hadn't been asked and that she would love to go with me. I absolutely can't remember a happier time at any time previous in my life.

Given it was my senior year, our conversation about marriage began within a couple months. I still had plans to attend Brigham Young University, even though I had no idea who Brigham Young was. Again, it was my fascination with BYU QBs throwing five to six touchdown passes per game that had me wanting to attend. But for various reasons, I wasn't living by the standards of BYU at the time, and instead I chose the University of Utah. Besides, my dad was still living there, and I could pick up on being a help to him too.

Later that summer, despite her being a strong Catholic girl and me being a semi-Mormon, Nancy and I were married. We chose a simple wedding service and had a wonderful reception that virtually the entire town was invited to. Nancy's mother, Joan, who was concerned about her daughter marrying a Mormon, nevertheless was supportive of us and has been a cherished person in our lives ever since. As I often tell her, I will never be able to repay her for her kindness, help, and unconditional love. I cried with great joy when I first saw her come in to my hospital bedside, thinking of her traveling many miles to be next to me at such a critical moment some thirty-seven years after meeting. I thought warmly of how much I owed her for her devoted love—and for allowing me to have Nancy's hand in marriage.

Chapter 10:

Celebrity Encounters

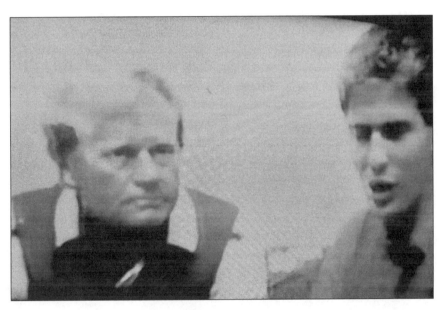

Jack Nicklaus

A live TV interview from Bigfork, Montana with former PGA star Jack Nicklaus two weeks after the "Golden Bear's" final Major win (MASTERS - May of 1986). In spite of the poor picture quality, it holds special meaning to me as it was a snapshot taken off her TV by my dear grandmother, Maybelle, as she watched the actual broadcast from her home in Anaconda.

O NE OF THE MOST EXCITING AND ENJOYABLE parts of being a television sportscaster and entertainment reporter for thirty years has been having the unique opportunity to meet famous athletes, acclaimed pop stars, and even the second man ever to walk on the moon all up close. From John

Stockton to Karl Malone, Muhammad Ali to Michael Jordan, or even Marie Osmond to Bill Murray, I've relished the opportunity to personally speak to them one on one—and always came away with a unique perspective of who they really were when the lights and cameras were turned off. I also recall interesting exchanges I had with them that shone a light on different perspectives of themselves—and me.

Jack Nicklaus

Back in 1986 Jack Nicklaus was known as the greatest golfer in PGA history—and most knowledgeable fans will tell you he still is today. That year, in what would be his world record eighteenth Majors title, the Golden Bear won the Masters Golf Championship in Augusta, Georgia, at the ripe old age of forty-six. I watched it all in amazement from my television in Kalispell, Montana. So imagine how much more I was amazed two weeks later when I was notified that Nicklaus himself would be making a special guest appearance at the Eagle Bend Gold Course in Bigfork, Montana, and that I was invited to come meet him! Just two years into my first TV sportscaster job, and I had the chance of a lifetime to interview the world's greatest golfer on live television.

My teeth chattered as I sat next to him, feverishly trying to think of legitimate questions for offer golf's all-time superstar. I guess I assumed he would be self-consumed with all his unprecedented fame, fortune, and success. However, in what turned out to be the greatest part of that day, I found Nicklaus to be extremely down-to-earth and the very definition of a consummate gentleman. As a proven veteran, he clearly must have recognized me as a young, nervous, and clearly exuberant reporter who was borderline giddy about this opportunity. But instead of impatiently behaving like he was above it all, Jack graciously answered all of my questions and showed me great dignity. Toward the end, he even took the time to compliment me on the job I did.

Ratings-wise and otherwise, that interview proved to be a huge success, thanks to the Golden Bear. Later that year it helped me become the Montana TV Broadcaster of the Year and set my career on a path of success that I will always be thankful for.

The other interesting lifelong lesson I received from Jack was a comment he made while we were visiting alone following the interview. I told him I had a bit of a kooky, personal question to ask, and he said I was free to ask him anything. "Well then, can you give me some indication of what it is like to be the greatest golfer in the world? The most loved and probably the richest?" As I asked that, I couldn't believe I had the nerve to. Still, in characteristic Jack Nicklaus form, his honest and forthright answer both stunned me and also helped me immensely in my life's journey. "You know," Jack said humbly, "I don't find any of those things to really be a big deal any more. The truth is, I'm looking for other things to do with my life at this point." I couldn't believe it! I mean, hundreds of thousands of us golfed each day hoping to be Jack Nicklaus, and yet, even if you ever did reach his status, it's not that big of a deal? It dawned on me at that very moment that perhaps many of us were wasting too much of our valuable earthly time chasing false dreams that, at best, would be fleeting.

Kurt Rambis and Michael Cooper

Just a year after the Nicklaus interview, I had another rare opportunity for a young TV journalist. Three weeks after the Los Angeles Lakers defeated the Boston Celtics for the NBA championshipo, I learned that two of the starting members of that Lakers team would be traveling to Ronan, Montana, of all places, to conduct a basketball camp for kids all across the state. Kurt Rambis and Michael Cooper were household names at that point, so I made the proper calls and wound up getting an exclusive opportunity to interview them. As I made the hour drive with my news photographer, I kept asking myself, "Is this really happening?" I mean, Ronan was a tiny, fairly obscure town in western Montana with a population of less than 2,000. How was it that these two stars would be there?

Yet as we pulled up and entered the gymnasium where the camp was being held, there they were. Two tall NBA stars tend to stand out in the crowd. I waited my turn as they finished drills with the kids, and then harnessed the gumption to ask them for a few minutes of their time. Not only did they agree, but they also made my year by inviting me to play them in a game of one-one-two! The hundreds of kids laughed and shouted joyously as the two stars schooled me on the court all in great fun. Afterward, with the camera still rolling, we had a pretend interview session where those two jokesters turned the tables by interviewing me. It was a dream come true for a young broadcaster, and somehow I had the feeling that they recognized my youth and need for help, and they reached out and gave it to me in a spectacular way.

Some fifteen years later, I came full circle with Rambis when, now as a major market reporter on FOX13 in Salt Lake City, I had the opportunity to meet up again with him while covering a Utah Jazz game against his Lakers. By this time, Rambis was the team's assistant head coach under Phil Jackson. Now more confident, but still a bit in awe of Rambis, I approached him after the game in the locker room and just had to ask, "Kurt, my name is Joe Wren. Do you happen to recall..." Before I could even finish the question, Rambis said, "That was *you*?" We both broke out in laughter and happily congratulated each other on our respective rises to success

John Stockton and Karl Malone

The year 1997 was by all accounts the greatest season to date for the NBA Utah Jazz. They finished the season with by far the best record in the Western Conference, thanks to future Hall of Famers John Stockton and Karl Malone. As the regular season came to a close, I was at both the team's games and their practices for postgame interviews. During that time I got to know them both very well. Both had world-caliber work ethic, and both were loyal to each other. It turned out they were also loyal to those in the media who were honest and genuine enough with them to treat them fairly journalistically. I always tried to be that guy, and one day John repaid me by doing something that I never heard of him doing for anyone before or since. Known for being a full-fledged recluse when it came to doing interviews, he openly admitted he only did them because the NBA and the Jazz required a certain amount of comments from him. But rather than dislike his behavior toward the media, I found it very refreshing. After all, here was a man of integrity who didn't consider himself above the game. Stockton was there simply to play and win.

Later, in one of the personal highlights of my professional career, John broke the stunning news of his impending retirement from basketball to me in the Jazz locker room. Hoards of reporters flooded over to where John and I were standing when they caught wind of it. *Sports Illustrated* and other national sports magazines actually printed the very question I asked him, as well as John's response.

Karl Malone was also staunchly loyal to those who he felt deserved it. While I never approached him on-court when they would warm up for a game, on several occasions Karl voluntarily came over to me and began conversations. He was, next to Michael Jordan, *the* biggest name in the NBA at the time, so I felt it was quite an honor. But rarely did he ever talk basketball to me. In fact, on one occasion he told me all about how he hunted wild hogs in Arkansas—and even invited me to come down during the off-season and try it out myself! On another occasion I was honored to find out that he was a fan of mine when I filled in on the FOX *Good Day Utah* morning show as an entertainment reporter.

Years later, when Jazz Owner Larry H. Miller passed away, Karl and his wife made a special trip up to the funeral at the Delta Center. I told my news director at FOX13 that I had a hunch he would do an interview with me if I just hung out with a photographer before he arrived. Sure enough, Karl eventually arrived, and would you believe he actually came right up to me and told me if he was to do any interview, it would be with me! As we began, several other media sources, including KSL's veteran star reporter John Hollenhorst, rushed up to get in on the interview, only to have Karl tell them, "No, this is the only person I am giving an interview to." I'd always respected and appreciated the positive way Karl portrayed the state of Utah in his words and actions, and now I was especially grateful to him for his loyalty.

Muhammad Ali

I had to pinch myself many times in June 1997. That was the month of the unforgettable, first-ever NBA Finals for the Utah Jazz. Only a few days before, I sat courtside in Houston as the Jazz pulled a stunning fifteen-point fourth-quarter comeback to defeat Charles Barkley and the Rockets in the West Conference Finals. That allowed them to advance to the World Finals against Michael Jordan and the Chicago Bulls.

As if traveling to Chicago for the Michael Jordan–primed Finals wasn't enough, I found out that I would be making the trip with former Jazz head coach Tom Nissalke. I remembered watching Tom coach when I caught an occasional game with my wife, Nancy, at the old Salt Palace. I was extremely proud to fly over with him—and found he was a hero in the Windy City. We arrived late on a Sunday night, and he insisted that we go to one of his favorite restaurants for stuffed pork chops. They were terrific, and so was he.

The first game wouldn't be until Wednesday night, but it was well worth waiting for. In fact, before the ball was even tossed up for Game 1, I was able to meet the man who would do the "tossing." I'd heard a rumor that former heavyweight boxing champion Muhammad Ali would be the man honored to take part in that opening toss, so I kept my eyes open for a first glimpse of him.

Since all of the media was taken care of like kings there, I decided to leave my cushy seat for a few moments to head up the corridor for a pregame meal. On my way up the aisle, there he was. He stood about 6'3", but he may as well have been 7'11". As a big fan of pro boxing growing up, I recognized Muhammad Ali immediately. Though he was suffering some of the effects of Parkinson's Disease, which he had contacted some ten years earlier, his eyes still had the same intensity and excitement that carried him through such world-renowned victories as the Thrilla in Manilla over "Smokin'" Joe Frazier and the shocking win over George Foreman in what was dubbed the "Rumble in the Jungle."

Ali had a bodyguard by his side, helping him make the walk down to the old Chicago Stadium. As I approached, I asked

50

Ali's aid if I could "shake hands with the Champ." Immediately Ali stepped toward me and made a championship fist as he smiled broadly. Clearly, though his body was shaking, his mind was clear and he was still eager to portray what he'd always referred to himself as: the Greatest. I was very pleased by his positive and caring personality. He knew I was from Utah, representing the Jazz, and he was enthusiastic about that too. I came away with an even more positive impression of the man than I had before.

Amazingly, I somehow was given a courtside media pass seat for that game—and actually sat next to ESPN host Dan Patrick. Ironically, just a week before I'd received a book in the mail called *The Big Show*, which chronicled the wild life behind the scenes of the networks highly rated sports program at the time by the same name. I brought that book with me to Chicago and carried it everywhere in my media backpack to read during breaks. So when I had the unique opportunity of showing it to Dan, he was very excited and immediately offered to sign the copy for me. I was now riding about as high as I could! So high that when I later showed it to then–Jazz VP David Allred that night, he asked to borrow it to read, and I let him. To date, he still hasn't returned it. I'm still waiting, David… Ha ha!

As a side note, during one of the off-days between games at the Finals that summer, I made my way to Chicago's Wrigley Field and secured a press pass to see the Cubs' game against the Pittsburgh Pirates from the field.

At the time, the Cubs were popular but not very good. One of the reasons for the team's popularity was found in their storied TV broadcaster, the incomparable Harry Caray. I took a gamble that night before the game and asked Harry if he would be willing to do a live interview with me. I had very little reason to believe he would, busy as I figured he was, but he did! In fact, it turned into one of the most hilarious interviews I'd ever done. The aging Caray was in full form, even suggesting that he loved Salt Lake City and followed me on-air when he was in town. I couldn't imagine most of the things he said to be true, but it was so funny and crazy that I went along with all of it.

Sadly, Caray passed away the following winter.

Charles Barkley

During the two-year NBA Finals run of the Jazz in 1997 and 1998, I had many opportunities to greet some of the greatest names in pro basketball. I shook hands with Magic Johnson at the Old Forum in Los Angeles during Utah's second-round series in '97 after having somehow made my way into the Lakers' top brass party shortly after Game 3.

But in Game 5 of the Western Conference Finals, I had a fun exchange with legendary Hall of Fame player and now TV analyst Charles Barkley. A couple hours after the Jazz had won the game to take a series lead of three games to two, I spotted Barkley and a young lady friend of his leaving the locker room.

I found him to be as personable as he is on TV; in fact, he offered to sign a Barkley basketball card I had brought to show him in case we had an opportunity to meet. I quickly accepted his offer of a signature. Unfortunately, the only pen I had was a felt tip, and after he signed it and handed it back, I gently squeezed it into the plastic covering that I brought it in. However, that squeeze was enough to smear his handwriting on the still-wet card. I didn't say anything, but as he watched me he could tell something was wrong. "You *smudged* it, didn't ya?" Charles asked me in his usual on-air tone. I said, "Yep." We both laughed, and he happily took the card back and signed the other side. I was pleased at how funny and patient he was.

I later donated that card to a charity fund-raiser, and I believe it brought in more than one hundred dollars.

Marie Osmond

Another highlight I enjoyed as a TV sportscaster for FOX13 came during the 2002 Winter Olympics in Salt Lake City. One of my assignments during the lead-up to the games was to cover the Olympic Torch as it made its way through the state of Utah before reaching Olympic Stadium in Salt Lake City. For three hours each morning, I had the grand opportunity of covering it live at a new venue during that final week leading up to the games. Just when it seemed the spectacular scenic shots couldn't get better, they did! From a stunning sunrise at

Arches National Park near Moab to a packed stadium of fans watching the torch take a lap around the stadium in Cedar City, I relished the overwhelming delight and pride the citizens of Utah took in hosting such a successful and worldwide event.

On the third morning, as the torch made its way to the American Fork area, I was assigned to do live shots from a car dealership just off I-15. Celebrities were generally present at every stop that I did broadcasts from, but on this occasion, I had a special live, impromptu guest.

In the middle of my live report on how positively the torch was being supported and appreciated by the thousands of fans around me, none other than Marie Osmond came up to me and gave me a great big, exuberant hug! She also made it clear how thrilled she was to be a part of the event, and how patriotic it felt to have such a huge turnout at every torch site.

The joy and happiness of finally having the world come to Salt Lake City was infectious, and so was Marie's personality and enthusiasm. I loved it, the gathered crowd loved it, and her unscripted appearance made that show one of the highest-rated morning shows of the year in Utah.

Bill Murray and Cheryl Ladd

I've followed former PGA star Johnny Miller's golf success ever since he shot a historic 63 at the U.S. Open back in 1973. No one had ever done it before, and it made him one of the top golfers in the world behind Jack Nicklaus for a couple years. Almost as much as I enjoyed watching his stylish and confident play, I grew to enjoy him as the best TV golf analyst ever. So when I learned he was hosting a celebrity golf tournament at Thanksgiving Point in Lehi back in 2006, I jumped at the opportunity to cover it.

True to form, Johnny gave me an excellent interview right on the golf course prior to the tee-off. His cool, relaxed, and knowledgeable style came off just as I'd hoped it would. I remain today one of his biggest fans, extremely impressed by how someone can move to world-class status in two different competitive professions.

Among the guest golfers was iconic comic Bill Murray, who hilariously kept the crowd in laughter simply by walking onto the course and teeing up his first ball. Some guys are so funny, and have such a rich history of comedic brilliance in the movies and on TV, that their mere presence garners adulation.

Former *Charlie's Angels* star Cheryl Ladd also had that adulation, though for other reasons than Murray. Back in 1977, Ladd had replaced the suddenly famous Farrah Fawcett on the show, and quickly gained superstardom herself portraying lovely and talented Kris Munroe on the hit series.

Few young men at the time will forget the poster of Cheryl that came out around that time. It sold millions and made her wel-known across the world. While I didn't have one myself growing up in Anaconda, most of my friends did. And when I mentioned during the live interview that some of my friends *still* have that poster, she jokingly said, "I've grown up, and now they need to, too!" She was classy and clearly eager to get rid of her sex-appeal image, which I respected very much.

Buzz Aldrin

While 1969 turned out to be a memorable year for me, U.S. astronaut Buzz Aldrin was clearly many moons beyond anything I would accomplish. As the entire world watched breathlessly, Aldrin joined fellow astronaut Neil Armstrong to become the planet's first two humans to walk on the moon. As the pilot aboard the lunar module on that historic Apollo 11 space mission, Buzz immediately followed Armstrong to set foot on the moon on July 21 at precisely 03:15:16.

Some thirty years later, Buzz landed next to me in what I found to be a momentous live interview from New York City. I was flown there to interview this famous man and to find out what made him tick. The interview itself, though fairly straightforward in terms of information we already knew, was fascinating. Listening to his every word, I followed up on the specifics of the mission itself. "While you and the rest of the world were watching the incredible live television broadcast from a place none of us had ever been to, or even saw up close before, I was totally absorbed in the highly complicated task or

54

landing us, fulfilling our many assignments while we were on the moon, and then somehow following every step NASA had planned out to ensure that we could get back safely," Aldrin told me. "To be honest, when I first went back to see the film that you all had already watched live, I didn't remember anything at all except for the specific instructions I had to perform and complete my duties, so watching it like that was as much fun for me as it was for the rest of the world when they originally saw it!"

I sat mesmerized as he calmly explained the overwhelming technical challenges Apollo 11 faced. Rather than having the luxury of utilizing advancements in modern science to ensure success on their unprecedented mission, their relatively rudimentary spacecraft was simply the impetus and forerunner to all the superior electronic technology that would be produced in the many decades that have since transpired. Essentially, Aldrin could see in hindsight that their success in such an incredible and successful journey was miraculous at the time.

As the interview wrapped up, I thanked him profoundly for reliving that singular event for us, and we parted ways.

Later that night, however, something very fortuitous allowed me to revisit that lunar landing. As I was walking past a lounge at the hotel we both were staying at, I noticed Aldrin sitting alone inside. While I'm not one to spend much time in taverns, I couldn't resist the idea of landing one more time next to Buzz. Intent on keeping my well-rehearsed ad-lib moment of salutation brief before my taking off, I was overjoyed to learn that this grand gentleman of space, Buzz Aldrin, would enthusiastically welcome me to join him. He knew I was from Utah, and while we didn't speak of specific religions, he did get quite religious in our conversation, to my great joy. In fact, I encouraged him to give me his insight on a very personal level of how that remarkable journey affected him from a spiritual perspective.

"I don't often speak of the spiritual side of that journey for me, but I can assure you there was one," Buzz opened up to me. I sat stargazing as these new thoughts were, to me, every bit as extraordinary and exciting as the earlier live interview— only these unique thoughts were so exclusive that the public had rarely ever heard them before.

"In one of the few opportunities of time I took while standing on the moon, I stared back at what, in essence, was a full Earth. Yes, I marveled at where I was in the universe, and at once I felt very small in proportion. However, I can also say that as I stood there, I received an overwhelming knowledge that God in heaven does exist. It was the most spiritual time I can remember."

I was blown away. I also came away with a strong knowledge that not only was Buzz Aldrin a supreme hero for the nation, and indeed the world, but he was also a champion of a human being in whom the Lord clearly saw fit to be honored with such a historic achievement. I was, and continue to be, very proud to have met him.

These days, now pushing ninety years old, a still strong, energetic, and science-conscious Aldrin continues to look toward the stars in the heavens. He recently took part in a virtual-reality holographic tour of the red planet in a film titled *Buzz Aldrin: Cycling Pathways to Mars*. A visually impressive movie highlighted by amazing imagery of the Martian landscape through new technology that features impressive and realistic holograms. The ten-minute film offers a realistic tour of the red planet, as well as a recreation of his firsthand encounter of being on the moon as one of his stops. Buzz said it was all about inspiring NASA to strongly consider one great master plan to pave a way for humans to one day settle on Mars. The year 2021 will be critical for any possible travel to Mars; in that year, the Earth and the red planet will align geographically to make travel there much easier than normal. Many other countries are also considering travel to Mars during that particular time.

Steve Young

Far and away the most admired pro sports figure I ever interviewed was Hall of Famer Steve Young. Young was always courteous, gracious, and straightforward—all while being a Super Bowl MVP–caliber quarterback.

I met him at several different locations, and each time, except the last, he was always upbeat, positive, and willing to take time for whatever questions I might have. He too was great at signing football cards, which my two sons loved. Our first visit was actually at an LDS ward in Kalispell. Steve put on a fireside up there the weekend he took part in a celebrity skiing event at Big Mountain in Whitefish in December 1989.

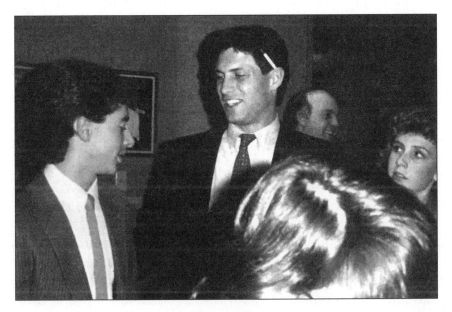

Steve Young

Years later, I took my oldest son, Matt, with me for one glorious sports weekend in September 1996. I was to work three games in two days, beginning with an MLB game featuring the Oakland A's on a Saturday afternoon, followed by a Utah vs. Stanford night game at Palo Alto. We would then make our way over to San Francisco to cover the Steve Young–powered 49ers.

Young was actually injured in that game, so it put a damper on our locker room meeting after the Niners' 37–0 rout of the St. Louis Cardinals. Nevertheless, true to form, Steve answered questions and manned up about the injury. Later I slipped him a note about his strong testimony and example to me. I noticed him read it as I walked out, and he turned to give me a smile and a thumbs-up.

Michael Jordan

While Steve Young was the professional star I most admired after meeting, Michael Jordan continues to be the biggest exclusive ever. (Yes, I've interviewed LeBron James, but I didn't find him to have near the charisma and magnitude of M.J.) While I would have loved to have had a one-on-one interview with Jordan back during the two NBA Finals against the Jazz, the truth is no one received those. After each game then, after all the media would flock into the locker room for postgame player interviews, M.J.'s superstar status allowed him to walk past us and into a large room where all the media would ask questions of him together. He was too big for the media, and we all recognized it.

But then one serendipitous afternoon near Tooele, Utah, I had the very coveted opportunity to meet and interview Jordan one-on-one exclusively for FOX13. As a veteran reporter, and after having been tipped off by Jazz owner Larry H. Miller (whom I loved) that Jordan would be there, I contacted M.J.'s PR person to formally request an interview. She had me send a fax describing my credentials, etc. Within a day she called me back and let me know they had decided to allow one Utah media person to interview Michael, and that was me!

I was so excited that I guess some of it poured out onto the court during my church basketball game that night. In my very vain attempts to emulate M.J., I suspect I became a little overly aggressive in my play. So much so that an opposing player gave me a rather vicious elbow that landed directly on my forehead and dropped me to the ground. As I came to, I noticed a great deal of blood pouring from the wound. Some of the guys rushed me to McKay Dee Hospital in Ogden, where a plastic surgeon gave me twenty-two stitches. About all I could think of was how this might affect my interview with Jordan.

The next morning was Wednesday. I woke up to peek into the mirror to see how badly my stitches and subsequent bruising was. To my delight, the stitching was done so well you could hardly notice it, and there was little or no bruising on my face. Since the interview wasn't until the next day, Thursday, it appeared I had dodged a bullet. However, come Thursday morning when I woke up, virtually the entire area of my cheek-bones below both eyes was as black as coal. I was devastated but still insisting on doing the interview. After all, I was the only one credentialed to do it, and no one else, even from FOX13, was allowed in.

My game plan for the interview was simple: since it was an outdoor event at Larry Miller's Motor Speedway, where Jordan's motorcycle race team was competing, I would simply wear sunglasses the whole time. It was a ploy that worked right up until just after the final question. As we were both standing to go our separate ways, Michael asked me, "Hey, nice interview... but what's with the sunglasses?" I then lifted the glasses up and told him that I had been injured a couple nights before playing basketball. He then said with a sly grin, "Hey, you're about my age... probably time for you to retire from basketball too!"

M.J. really impressed me by being extremely articulate and using great wisdom with every word he spoke. He also took me over to his trailer after and gave me Michael Jordan headbands, wristbands, and even M.J. bottled water. A real class act.

LeBron James

LeBron Raymone James, perhaps better known as King James in the sporting world, may be the best player ever in the NBA—or the world, for that matter. He was a first-round draft pick right out of high school who has since won three NBA championships, four NBA MVP Awards, three NBA Finals MVP Awards, a pair of Olympic gold meals, and a host of other individual and All-Star awards—all while supposedly still being in his prime. Not bad for a child who grew up with a single mother in a very tough area of Akron, Ohio. Right now he is said to be worth around $350 million, with hundreds of millions coming from endorsements. Ironically, though he grew up without many family members by his side, one of his early TV endorsements stirred a topic that got him to open up to me following a game his Cleveland Cavaliers played against the Utah Jazz in Utah back in January 2009. While the rising star was still in his elementary stages of pro basketball, James showed plenty of charm and personality during a series of commercials he starred in for Nike around that time.

Following a hard-fought five-point Cavs win, I did a live report courtside for FOX13 TV. Afterward, I immediately walked back in to get an up-close glimpse of LeBron in Cleveland's postgame locker room. Since FOX13's early news begins an hour earlier than the other stations in Salt Lake City, I generally had the players to myself for interviews while the other sports guys in town were busy on-air.

On this occasion, I could tell LeBron was understandably worn-out and tired from not only the game but also from giving interviews that night. He begrudgingly answered a few easy questions from me and then appeared eager to dismiss me when a thought suddenly came to my head. Earlier that week I recalled laughing with my sons about his hilarious TV ads, and with that still on my mind, I blurted out to LeBron, "Got a good laugh at that new Nike commercial where you played your dad and brothers." He immediately popped his head back up as his demeanor transitioned to a full-court smile as he excitedly replied, "Yeah, you like those too?" His countenance changed delightedly as he told me briefly about how they made them and then said, "If you like those, I have an even better one coming out in a couple of weeks." After shaking hands and walking off, I was happy not only to see a unique side of him but to be able to say something that would bring a little happiness into his life. His smile was real, and so was mine.

Chapter 11:

President Kimball

WHILE THE WORLDLY FUN OF INTERVIEWING famous celebrities has always provided great thrills of excitement, as life rolled on, I became more interested in seeking those things that offer great meaning to why we are all here on earth and where it is that we are all going. There are obviously many misconceptions about the Church of Jesus Christ of Latter-Day Saints. Though polygamy, which was established originally by God in the Old Testament, hasn't been practiced by the Church of Jesus Christ of Latter-Day Saints members since the 1800s, a recent poll suggests more than one-quarter of Americans still believe the religion practices it.

I remember even as a boy at St. Paul's Junior High hearing one of my English teachers making fun of the LDS faith. At the time, I was just starting to attend so I was disheartened that a teacher, of all people, would be spreading ideas that I knew even then were untrue. Still, I could see how there could be many false thoughts or ideas from anyone who superficially knew and spoke of the religion.

Many have described, possibly in attempts to seduce fellow parishioners into fear, the LDS Church as a cult. A potentially effective slander—partly because, at least for me, that term always seemed to conjure up devilish images, specifically designed as such by those hoping to discredit the faith as evil. The dictionary describes the word *cult* as "a relatively small group of people having religious beliefs or practices regarded by others as strange or sinister."

Well, guess what? By that same standard, the Savior Himself, Jesus Christ, may also have been described as leading a cult. His mortal ministry was small and clearly different from the predominant but false religions of the time. Yet when the Only Begotten Son of God finally came into this world, those prideful Jewish priests chose to call Him false names, ridicule Him, shun Him, lie about Him, tortured Him, and eventually murder Him on the cross.

They did so because they claimed he spoke disrespectfully or irreverently of God and sacred things. Many times Jesus Christ was charged with speaking blasphemy because he claimed the right to forgive sins.

> Matthew 9: 2–3 "They also hated the Savior in the name of their skewed interpretation of 'religion' because He dared call himself the Son of God."

> John 10: 22–36 "And it was at Jerusalem the feast of the dedication, and it was winter. And Jesus walked in the temple in Solomon's porch. Then came the Jews round about him, and said unto him, How long dost thou make us to doubt? If thou be the Christ, tell us plainly. Jesus answered them, I told you, and ye believed not: the works that I do in my Father's name, they bear witness of me. But ye believe not, because ye are not of my sheep, as I said unto you. My sheep hear my voice, and I know them, and they follow me: And I give unto them eternal life; and they shall never perish, neither shall any man pluck them out of my hand. My Father, which gave them me, is greater than all; and no man is able to pluck them out of my Father's hand. I and my Father are one. Then the Jews took up stones again to stone him. Jesus answered them, Many good works have I shewed you from my Father; for which of those works do ye stone me? The Jews answered him, saying, For a good work we stone thee not; but for blasphemy; and because that thou, being a man, makest thyself God.

Jesus answered them, Is it not written in your law, I said, Ye are gods? If he called them gods, unto whom the word of God came, and the scripture cannot be broken; Say ye of him, whom the Father hath sanctified, and sent into the world, Thou blasphemest; because I said, I am the Son of God?"

I've often wondered how it is that Jesus Christ Himself, the Lord and Redeemer of everyone who has ever lived or anyone who yet will live, could be so misjudged by the supposed top religious minds of the time. To be honest, I feel a similar way to that today about the Church of Jesus Christ of Latter-Day Saints. Plenty of misconceptions may be keeping many from enjoying the endless feelings of joy that are out there.

The entire New Testament testifies of the divinity of Jesus Christ today, yesterday, and tomorrow. Jesus was the first person to be resurrected on earth. By overcoming death, He set the path for every other person born on earth to also be resurrected.

> Acts 26:23 "That Christ should suffer, and that he should be the first that should rise from the dead, and should shew light unto the people..."

To fully emphasize that He *was* resurrected and did, in fact, receive the glorified body that He promised He would, Jesus even returned and arose with that physical body. Amazingly, not only was His tomb empty, He ate fish and honey *after* His mortal death! The New Testament tells that Christ showed His body of flesh and bones to hundreds of people. They came up to Him and were allowed to touch Him while the angels testified that He had risen, even after His crucifixion, to unquestionably testify to all that He had become what He promised He would.

> John 20: 1–18 "The first day of the week cometh Mary Magdalene early, when it was yet dark, unto the sepulchre, and seeth the stone taken away from the sepulchre. Then she runneth, and cometh to Simon Peter, and to the other disciple, whom Jesus loved, and saith unto them, They have taken away the Lord out of the sepulchre,

> and we know not where they have laid him. Peter therefore went forth, and that other disciple, and came to the sepulchre. So they ran both together: and the other disciple did outrun Peter, and came first to the sepulchre. And he stooping down, and looking in, saw the linen clothes lying; yet went he not in. Then cometh Simon Peter following him, and went into the sepulchre, and seeth the linen clothes lie. And the napkin, that was about his head, not lying with the linen clothes, but wrapped together in a place by itself. Then went in also that other disciple, which came first to the sepulchre, and he saw, and believed.

"For as yet they knew not the scripture, that he must rise again from the dead. Then the disciples went away again unto their own home. But Mary stood without at the sepulchre weeping: and as she wept, she stooped down, and looked into the sepulchre, And seeth two angels in white sitting, the one at the head, and the other at the feet, where the body of Jesus had lain. And they say unto her, Woman, why weepest thou? She saith unto them, Because they have taken away my Lord, and I know not where they have laid him. And when she had thus said, she turned herself back, and saw Jesus standing, and knew not that it was Jesus.

"Jesus saith unto her, Woman, why weepest thou? whom seekest thou? She, supposing him to be the gardener, saith unto him, Sir, if thou have borne him hence, tell me where thou hast laid him, and I will take him away. Jesus saith unto her, Mary. She turned herself, and saith unto him, Rabboni; which is to say, Master. "Jesus saith unto her, Touch me not; for I am not yet ascended to my Father: but go to my brethren, and say unto them, I ascend unto my Father, and your Father; and to my God, and your God. Mary Magdalene came and told the disciples that she had seen the Lord, and that he had spoken these things unto her."

So how is it that the Church of Jesus Christ of Latter-Day Saints is now the only religion on earth that understands and fully believes that Jesus *still* has a resurrected body that was the entire focal point of the Bible? Nowhere in scripture does it claim anything else.

Sadly, the answer to why most religions now teach that Jesus is no longer the resurrected man he told us about can be traced back to the year 325 AD, several hundred years after Jesus's death. At that time, in the city of Nicea and without direct revelation from God, instead solely based on the flawed beliefs of religious leaders at the time who sharply disagreed on many issues of the Church, a man-made determination was made that henceforth all religions would teach that Jesus Christ no longer had a resurrected body. This was commonly known as the Nicean Creed.

And there you have it. The entire Biblical objective of our Lord and Savior was to show us unquestionably that He would gain a resurrected body, which He did and promised us that so will we. This objective was inexplicably changed and dramatically distorted simply to fit the purposes and false narratives of man, not the Lord.

> Luke 24: 36–43 "And as they thus spake, Jesus himself stood in the midst of them, and saith unto them, Peace be unto you. But they were terrified and affrighted, and supposed that they had seen a spirit. And he said unto them, Why are ye troubled? and why do thoughts arise in your hearts? Behold my hands and my feet, that it is I myself: handle me, and see; for a spirit hath not flesh and bones, as ye see me have.

"And when he had thus spoken, he shewed them his hands and his feet. And while they yet believed not for joy, and wondered, he said unto them, Have ye here any meat? And they gave him a piece of a broiled fish, and of an honeycomb. And he took it, and did eat before them."

Nowhere in the Bible will you read that Jesus Christ no longer has a glorified body; in fact, quite the opposite. The entire purpose of the Church of Jesus Christ of Latter-Day Saints, revealed through a modern-day prophet—Joseph Smith—is to reinstall the truth, direct from the Savior himself, that He lives and has a glorified body. Thus, as the scriptures clearly note, we join Jesus Christ as being fellow children of God the Eternal Father. And as His children, God the Eternal Father has effectively assured us that we are each heirs to all that He has—meaning everything there is or ever was.

> Romans 8:17 "And if children, then heirs; heirs of God, and joint-heirs with Christ; if so be that we suffer with him, that we may be also glorified together."

Unquestionably, meeting some of the world's most famous athletes and Hollywood celebrities has provided me numerous worldly thrills and even a few great life lessons. Yet it seemed the more of them I met, the more I realized that despite their fame and fortune, there was a collective cap on just how much joy and happiness they could receive from their vaunted celebrity status. Ultimately, even if any of the rest of us were to reach that pinnacle of success in any particular field, eventually we would inevitably become dissatisfied with the finite limits we could reach and wind up still searching for true meaning to life.

The bottom line is even being the very best and most successful people on the planet in any particular field outside of true religion won't be enough to quench our innate drive to know who we are, where we came from, or where we are going.

About a year after Nancy and I were married, we were living on the upper east side of Salt Lake City in 1980. I had been accepted to the University of Utah, and we were living in the U's student housing along with our newborn son, Matthew. The addition of children to your home often seems to bring a sense of urgency for religious stabilization for parents. The realization of such a new and awesome responsibility, as is correct and appropriate, began to weigh on our minds and motivate us to forget a little of ourselves and begin to recognize our sacred duty to those for whom we had to make vital decisions in those critical early years.

Matthew 4:4 "He answered and said, it is written, Man shall not live by bread alone, but by every word that proceedeth out of the mouth of God."

Critical decisions for our children go beyond just food and housing into every physical, mental, and spiritual need they have. So as our marriage progressed, so did our discussions on religious faith. Oftentimes I would not only go with Nancy to the Catholic church in town, she would attend the LDS ward with me too. Afterward we would discuss the things we learned and what we believed, and sometimes didn't always believe, about what was being taught there. Our conversations would occasionally become argumentative, as we both had our points of view, but overall we recognized it as a good way of coming closer together, especially when done in a peaceful way that would invite the true spirit into our hearts and minds. The key factor for us turned out to be the nature of God the Father and Jesus Christ today. What does the Bible teach us about who they are? After reading that Moses spoke face-to-face with the God of this world, we were both convinced that the Lord, in fact, had a body and always will.

Exodus 33:11 "And the LORD spake unto Moses face to face, as a man speaketh unto his friend. And he turned again into the camp: but his ser- vant Joshua, the son of Nun, a young man, departed not out of the tabernacle."

Eventually we would meet many young, wonderful couples close to our age in the student housing "village" that we lived in. We found them to be some of the greatest people we'd ever known. Many of them had just served LDS church mis- sions and were eager and knowledgeable enough to discuss the things they'd learned with Nancy and I. Despite attending the Mormon Church for a few years, I had yet to fully read *The Book of Mormon* and frankly didn't know what it was about, and neither did Nancy. One of our friends in the housing, John Prince, actually had a younger brother who had been a "home teacher" to the current president of the LDS Church, Spencer

W. Kimball. A home teacher is one of two people who, as a tandem, briefly visit a few families in their ward area each month to check up on them and make sure they have all their needs met.

I'd heard a great deal around that time about President Kimball, and I was very, very interested in the possibility of personally meeting him one day. Knowing that it could also be a great benefit to Nancy to meet this prominent LDS Church leader, John notified me around that time that the church president would actually be giving a Christmastime talk in his own home ward, which was less than a mile from where we lived. We were delighted when he told us that we could both come with him as a guest to hear the talk. Both Nancy and I were thrilled at what we might learn, and quickly accepted. My excited anticipation grew greater and greater as the day of the talk grew near.

President Kimball was the only church leader I had ever known of since joining the LDS faith, and I carried full expectations of how great a religious moment it would be to see him, and I hoped I might even get a chance to personally meet him along the way. I was confident that the Lord had a hand in this opportunity, and therefore I was expecting something grand. Surely, I thought, meeting a convert like myself and knowing how many unlikely hurdles I'd already jumped to learn of the church would impress him.

Finally, the chilly December morning arrived that we would be able to meet the man I had heard so much of. I actually had butterflies in my stomach as I nervously anticipated seeing him and, Lord willing, speaking with him.

Being guests of John, he drove us to the church building and led the way into the chapel. My eyes searched and searched for the president as we walked in and found seats, but I couldn't see him anywhere. Finally, after sitting a few moments, I leaned over and curiously asked John if President Kimball was even there. He smiled and said, "Yes, as a matter of fact, you just walked right past him!"

My head turned quickly toward the entryway, and sure enough, there he was. I'd walked past him because I didn't recognize him. The irony wasn't lost on me. I suppose I was expecting someone who was physically larger than life, but I found him to be relatively frail and small. After all, he was eighty-five years old and had been dealing with serious health issues of a poor heart and throat cancer for years.

Without even thinking, I popped up and told Nancy that I needed to go meet him before the meeting began. I quickly walked to him, my heart beating faster and faster with each step. *I'm about to meet* President Kimball*, and he's about to meet* me, I thought to myself. As I arrived before him, I stretched out my hand with great pride and said, "President, my name is Joe Wren, and I've wanted to meet you for quite some time."

I was so proud of myself.

Honestly, though, in all of my thoughts about that moment, I hadn't ever even considered or anticipated what my plans would be from that point on. Still, somewhere in the back of my mind I guess I thought trumpeting angels might be in order. Perhaps a "hallelujah"? Neither occurred. In fact, to this day I remember something quite different than the pat on the back "Attaboy, Joe" I was awaiting. The kindly look on his face suddenly became stoic and serious, and I was confused. As he took my hand, it wasn't really what I'd call a "shake"; it was more of a "hold." And instead of a boisterous smile and glowing comments on how great it was to have me in the church, what a great guy I was, and how proud of me he was, he simply held on to my hand and stared at me as if he'd known me for a thousand years or much more. I grew slightly uncomfortable as he kept my hand for what seemed to be ten to fifteen seconds. I don't even remember him saying much besides, "It's good to have you here; welcome."

I have to say I was confused and even slightly offended. Here I was, in all my religious arrogance, expecting him to outpour a great deal of joy and affection toward me. But as I somberly returned to sit in the church pew and digest all of it, it seemed more like he'd just taken me to the ecclesiastical woodshed. Granted, I thought to myself, I wasn't perfect. While I was trying to attend church as much as I could, it's true that I wasn't living up to every standard. I had long hair, but it was in line with the current styles. And no, I didn't have the full sense of urgency for religion that our wonderful neighbors in the student family housing apartments did; I didn't even make it a habit of keeping the Sabbath Day holy, let alone having a constant prayer in my heart. Still, I was there, right?

The more I thought of it, the more bitter I started to become as I worked up unpleasant, prideful thoughts in my mind. I thought to myself, there I was, a fine person trying to do the right things in this increasingly unrighteous world. Shouldn't this man of God be grateful and jump for joy at my effort?

As the sacrament meeting came to an end with President Kimball's talk winding down, I have to admit I hadn't fully listened enough to concentrate and absorb all he had said. In my childish pouting, I'd spent more time thinking of the awful possibility that all I'd been through trying to make my way into the church these past eleven years may have been misguided. Through either shame or bitterness, I didn't even want to look up at him. But as he was drawing near on the final words of his talk, I felt impressed to look up as a new tone came about him and his countenance seemed to change somewhat.

His final words began, "And I want you all to know..." I sat up at that point and paid particular attention, because at that very moment he clearly placed his eyes on me out of the entire congregation as he completed his final thought. "I want you all to know that I love you." He looked at me and we made a clear connection. He was telling me, personally, in an honest and sincere way that he loved me.

Now I was really confused. How was it that just an hour after taking me to the woodshed, President Kimball was telling me that he loved me in a way so poignant and real that I could feel his deep love and appreciation for me all throughout my heart and mind?

> 1 Corinthians 13:11 "When I became a man, I put away childish things."

Immediately it came to me. Perhaps not having had a father around to properly discipline me to that point in my life enticed the Lord Himself to reserve this needed moment to impress upon me a sense of urgency to grow up and be a man. It was high time that I move forward with what the Lord wanted and needed from me instead of selfishly basking in a shallow and self-made glow. Through the man who originally coined the phrase "Just do it" many years before marketing wizards caught on to what a wonderfully positive message it is, I had just been taught a monumental lesson in shifting attention from my own vanity toward the ever-present needs of those around me. Forget yourself and help others.

Equally important was the reaction that Nancy had enjoyed via the Holy Spirit that day. As I was off learning lessons on humility, the spirit was teaching her divine lessons on the Holy Ghost. While she didn't mention anything at the time, I recognized that she'd spent the rest of the day considering the words of President Kimball and the feelings of peace and joy that accompanied them.

I recognized that she'd spent the rest of the day considering the words of President Kimball and the feelings of peace and joy that accompanied them, and later that night, when we were alone on a trip home from my grandmother's house, Nancy confided to me that she now wanted to be baptized into the Church of Jesus Christ of Latter-Day Saints.

Chapter 12:

The Cardston Temple Miracle

AROUND MY JUNIOR YEAR OF COLLEGE, NANCY
and I made a decision to return to Montana to complete
my education. At the University of Utah I was majoring in jour-
nalism with an emphasis on radio and television, and they
just happened to offer that same major at the University of
Montana in Missoula. Besides, we were eager to get back
closer to friends and relatives there—not to mention my finger-
prints had been nearly permanently removed from the hours
and hours of loading and unloading boxes at UPS to provide
a living for us there.

Shortly before leaving, we had the wonderful opportunity of
having our marriage sealed in the newly opened Jordan River
Temple. By then, Nancy had also given birth to a baby girl,
whom we named Jill. In the temple ceremony, both Jill and Matt
were walked into the sealing room to be sealed to us for time
and all eternity. It was truly one of the highlights of our young
lives, and the blessings of that day continue to compound for
us with each minute as we see our children having grown and
developed the grand talents the Lord has seen fit to instill in
them. The Holy Spirit was always strong and assuring as we
sought the Lord in leading us to lead them.

Through all the joy and happiness she felt spiritually, Nancy
had a difficult time discussing her baptism with her dear mother,
Joan. In all my life, I have rarely found a woman of such strength,
dignity, character, and love for her family as I did in Joan. Each
time I look at her, I can still recall the immense strength it must
have taken that day when she escorted her seven children
to the Sunnyside Cemetery in Anaconda to bury her beloved

husband, Fred. His premature death at age forty-four was as shocking as it was sad. Along with being a former teacher, principal, superintendent, and head coach, Fred was a hero in town for being a strong leader of his family of nine. While Joan has deep roots and strong tradition in her Catholic faith, she also recognizes the importance of supporting the decisions of faith Nancy has chosen, as best as she can. I believe it takes an incredible, Christlike person to be as loving and understanding as she was, and continues to be, even though seeing her oldest daughter convert wasn't what she'd intended to happen. Still, too many times to even recall, Joan would come to our aid in one form or another during those early years of our marriage. I know that the Lord loves her dearly and will make all things correct to her at a chosen time. I've always tried to keep Joan in my thoughts, prayers, and actions, as well as her late husband, Fred. I consider it a great honor and privilege to be a part of the amazing Moodry family that is now iconic in the city of Anaconda.

On our first day arriving in Missoula in early June 1982, I immediately went looking for a job. I'd been told that the employment situation in town was very limited, but I also felt like the Lord intended for me to be there. Before heading out, I prayerfully recognized the type of work I felt I'd like to pursue and benefit from the most, and then boldly walked in to seek employment at KPAX-TV. While this was the first TV station I'd ever been into, I can only presume the confidence I carried as I bounded in effectively made up for my overwhelming lack of experience, because by the time I'd left, the general manager had given me a job. It wasn't much, but it was a start, and I was promised more opportunities if I worked hard, learned the craft, and improved my abilities daily. Within a few months I was shocked to be offered a promotion to weekend news anchor—something I'd aspired to professionally since I was eleven years old. While covering sports was my primary objective, I certainly wasn't foolish enough to give up such an opportunity. Back in those days, believe it or not, they were just getting past film and into videotape for the presentation of the news highlights of the day. Now I was preparing to take a quantum leap of my own.

During that time, I also attended class full-time at the U of M, and even landed another part-time job at the local UPS location in Missoula. Anyone who works there can tell you that the work is very hard, but the pay is also very good.

Later that fall, for extra money and additional on-the-job training, I picked up another part-time job. Truth be told, this one was mainly for excitement and fun. I considered it more of an exciting recreation than vocation. With the 1982 college football season approaching, I met up with a good man, Bill Schwanke, who was referred to as the Voice of the Montana Grizzlies. At the time, Bill covered every U of M college football broadcast on the statewide radio network. Somehow I convinced him to allow me to be his sideline reporter for all the games. I also remember and appreciate him for caring enough and having enough faith in me to hire me. Shortly after the positive experience of that season, the competing TV station across town, KECI-TV, offered me the more coveted role as a weekend TV sports anchor.

While the whole adventure of winding up in the very professional workplace that I'd always dreamed of seemed almost too easy, I now look back at the professional pattern of my broadcasting career and can clearly see the Lord's hand, as every job I ever had in this profession would almost directly lead me to the next.

Within a year of working at KECI, I was informed that a full-time sports director position was opening at KCFW-TV in Kalispell, Montana. I still had more than a quarter of school remaining before graduation, but my family needed me to make more money. Besides, I was very eager and excited to get moving on my career. I applied and eventually received that job thanks to a kindly GM, Mike Stocklin. So in March 1984 I moved our young family to northern Montana and began my television sports career. By the time I was ready to move on from Kalispell five years later, I had won Montana TV Broadcaster of the Year twice and felt I prepared to move up to another challenge.

Even more important than my professional success in Kalispell, I found great personal and spiritual happiness. In 1987 our second son, Tyler, was born. For reasons known only to the Lord, and likely because Nancy was such a model person, we were blessed with another seemingly perfect child.

The other major blessing of that period occurred in 1986. Though I was working full-time, my salary in those days was a mere $1,000—not much considering I was trying to raise a family of five. Nancy made some extra money for us by occasionally babysitting for neighbors, and she even worked part-time in a pizza parlor owned by some of our friends for a year, but we still found ourselves hurting for money each month.

As any young, poor family can attest, being without finances can be a heavy burden to a marriage, as well as your overall happiness... if you allow it to be. For the most part, Nancy and I dedicated our humble lives to our beautiful children—and found the greatest of joy and happiness in them. As they attended primary Sunday school meetings, our hearts were filled with love and joy watching them sing and invite the feeling of the Lord into their own souls. Though still in infant stages ourselves of learning of the mysteries of God at that time, we knew we were very happy.

Mormon temples are now found throughout the world, and members with recommendations are encouraged to attend them as often as possible for blessings and spiritual strength. But in those days, temples weren't as plentiful as they are now, and our living nearly four hours from the nearest one, in another country, was problematic. The Cardston, Alberta, Temple in southern Canada was not only a long drive, it required a good deal of money that we simply didn't have for gas and expenses. However, one day in March 1986, a married couple in our Kalispell Third Ward let us know they were planning to attend the temple to be sealed and asked us if we would come attend. While it was a financial hardship that we had to scrimp and save for, somehow we both realized it was a very important thing to do.

Revelations 14:13 "Here are they that keep the commandments of God, and the faith of Jesus."

That day I would learn, in the strongest way possible, that if you keep the commandments of God, challenges notwithstanding, and live for your life on hope and faith that the Lord will provide great blessings, He will never let you down. And in fact, all that effort made for that trip would soon produce one of the two most incredibly spiritual moments of my life to this point.

As we loaded up the children, food, and various supplies in our car for an early departure that Saturday morning, March 29, my thoughts were almost exclusively focused on the long drive and how we might be able to cut a few corners financially. Ideally we would have had the money to stay overnight in a hotel, but the reality was that we could barely afford to drive up, attend a temple session that lasted about two hours, and then drive back home as soon as possible. Besides, we also needed extra money to pay a babysitter to watch Matthew and Jill, and since we'd rarely ever used a babysitter, we weren't even sure what that cost would be. Safe to say, especially in a day and age of not having GPS, it was about all Nancy and I could do to merely get our family to southern Alberta, Canada, let alone give it the deep, spiritual thought we should have. In fact, I hadn't even stopped to consider that it was Easter weekend. To me, given I was still somewhat in the elementary stages of religious knowledge, Easter in many ways still meant candy, eggs, and a furry rabbit. Nevertheless, the overwhelming significance of this most sacred of holidays would be forever impressed upon me by the time the afternoon was complete.

We'd previously made arrangements for a kindly local family in Cardston to tend to our kids during the few hours we would be at the temple. While dropping them off, we were comforted to find them very loving and caring. So with that, we were finally on our way to gain a first look at the original Mormon temple to be built outside of the United States of America.

At the time of its completion in 1923, this beautiful edifice was just the sixth temple in the world. At this writing, there are now 155, with fourteen more under construction and another eight announced. Each temple comes with its own unique exterior, and at nearly 82,000 square feet and 85 feet tall, this one took its physical inspiration from Solomon's Temple of old. As we neared it, we received a warm, spiritual feeling that had been absent during our wild rush to get there.

LDS faithful gather inside together, regardless of which ward or stake you attend in the world. Inside the temple parishioners attend a session together before exiting though a gloriously designed celestial room. Each of the temples are opened to the public prior to being dedicated, so anyone in the world can consider themselves cordially invited to come see them personally, and enjoy the architectural beauty that is there. "Not secret, just sacred."

> Jonah 2:7 "When my soul fainted within me I remembered the Lord: and my prayer came in unto thee, into thine Holy Temple."

The two-hour temple session was uplifting, as they always are. It also helped us restore the peace and serenity that had been missing the prior couple of days as we feverishly made our plans for travel. So as of that moment, I felt more peace and comfort but nothing extraordinary.

A marriage sealing is performed whenever a man and woman, formerly married, choose to make their union eternal, although generally they are made as part of their original marriage ceremony. When a sealing takes place, there is one additional gathering in temple. When sealed for "time and all eternity," there is a special room dedicated in which all who were invited by the couple are to meet. On this exceptional day, I was directed to go to a special meeting room to await the other male members of the group. The bishop of my ward in Kalispell joined me, and we arrived in there together; we were the first two there. Peacefully and quietly, we took our seats and both began to ponder and pray silently to ourselves.

Mere minutes passed when something extraordinary, unanticipated, and never before felt by me overcame my body, mind, and soul to my great amazement. I opened my eyes a time or two to see if it were something physical that was giving me such an "uplift." Seeing nothing was there, I went back to thoughtful prayer. But immediately after continuing meditation, the feeling roared back much stronger and with a spiritual power that I had never, ever previously known. Fully unprepared to receive such a compelling feeling, all I could do was sit mesmerized.

Joyfully and lovingly I was richly overwhelmed with an extremely deep feeling of both the existence and presence of God the Eternal Father and His Son, Jesus Christ—and everyone else in the world, for that matter. As tears flowed down my cheeks, I knew as sure as I was sitting there that the Savior lived and was much closer to me than I'd ever imagined.

Being so carried away in the Spirit, I hadn't \ given attention to or even noticed the bishop sitting beside me, or how he was reacting to my emotions. When I finally glanced over to him, it was abundantly clear that he too was receiving this identical immense spiritual gift. While I don't recall how long after it was from that moment, a member of the temple presidency then entered the door, silently walked in, and stood before us. As he did, it was plain and obvious to him that the two of us had experienced something very marvelous. His only words to us were, "I see that you recognize what has transpired here this weekend." So sacred are the everyday ceremonies of the temple sessions that I dare not say anything that isn't fully truthful.

To a much larger degree, in this case, I dare not go into great detail about what our conversation was, or even precisely why I was feeling the way I did. Nevertheless, our profound spiritual feelings that afternoon, though they really didn't need to be, were fully confirmed as coming directly from the Only Begotton Son of God the Eternal Father, through the Holy Ghost.

I walked out of that room with a stunningly new perspective on the world and the heavens. While I had spent many years learning and believing the teachings of the Church of Jesus Christ of Latter-Day Saints, it now dawned on me in an absolute and epic way that this visitation was a quantum leap above everything that I had ever known or felt before. My undeniable understanding now was that God the Father lives, as does his son, Jesus Christ. As a result, I personally witnessed that Christianity is true and real, as is the Bible and *The Book of Mormon*.

Jesus Christ truly did suffer in the Garden of Gethsemane and ultimately was tortured and died for each of us on the cross at Calvary. Our lives, including everyone who has ever lived or ever will live, personally and singularly matter to God the Father and to the Savior—so much so that they not only know and care about every thought we've ever had, but they also love us infinitely and eternally! They want us to live righteously, love one another, and return to a heavenly glory. They want us with them in that new estate, even after ultimate death from this mortal world, so that we can live in a fully wonderful and resurrected way of joy and happiness forever! Amen!

For weeks, I could barely think of anything else. Having been so caught off guard by it, I couldn't even fully put the experience into words at the time, and had no idea why a soul so unprepared and seemingly unworthy as mine could be gifted in such a way. I was slightly embarrassed knowing that I was a sinner, and that others were truly much, much better than me.

But I also recognized finally what the Lord meant in the scriptures when it was written:

> Deuteronomy 6:13 "Thous shalt fear the Lord they God…"

Many times previously in life I had wondered how it is that we should fear such a great and loving Father in heaven. But this experience immediately made it clear to me that the "fear" spoken of in Deuteronomy simply refers to that final day when we will all come before the Savior to be judged. We will be wise to fear the potentially awful shame and sorrow that will be ours standing before the great Jehovah, who was the only perfect one among us, and one who lived and died for us, having to express unrepented sins that will be like scarlet. Even so much as having told a lie will cause consternation.

> Deuteronomy 6:24 "Fear the Lord… for good always"

I hadn't even known of these scriptures in Deuteronomy prior to that eye-opening experience, so it gave me great contentment and assurance to go back and find the meaning of what they meant in Biblical context.

> Psalms 111–115 "Fear of the Lord is the beginning of wisdom… Blessed is the man that feareth the Lord… Ye that fear the Lord, trust in the Lord… Then thou shalt understand the fear of the Lord."

Only to close members of my family did I speak about this until years later—partially because of feeling I wasn't worthy of it and partially because of me trying to understand and make sense of it all. Similar to the great lesson President Kimball had taught me years earlier, I again had much to figure out in my mind and soul about exactly what lessons and purposes were meant for me. The one certain thing was that I knew that what I had felt and witnessed *was real and glorious*, and not even the thirty years since has dimmed that knowledge in any way, nor would I ever be so foolish as to deny it. The real question turned out to be, would I be able to sustain myself and live strictly according to the Lord's will forever because of it?

Chapter 13:

A New Challenge

WE LIVED HAPPILY AND JOYFULLY IN KALISPELL the next two and a half years. During that time, another incredible blessing occurred when our second son, Tyler, was born at Kalispell Regional Hospital. Tyler has been exquisitely wonderful ever since those first few seconds of his birth. He has great intelligence, talents, and a love for what is right—including his devotion to the Savior in his thoughts and actions.

Though I longed to further my career, in hindsight, those would be some of the best days of my life. We loved our children so, and even with very little money, we found ways of being together with them camping, going to parks, or simply taking long walks together. The testimony I received in the temple carried me like a warm coastal breeze. I loved life and those around me.

Then in early December 1988, I learned of a TV sports director job opening up in Butte, Montana. While it wouldn't be an enormous professional climb, I was immediately interested because Butte is less than a half hour away from Anaconda, and the opportunity to go back and cover sports each night before the very people I grew up with sounded very enticing. As each minute rolled by, my desire and enthusiasm for that job grew. Though Nancy immediately expressed concerns about the move, Kalispell is very pretty, and we had many friends there, not to mention the very positive steps we'd taken in the gospel and with our family.

She made very good points, but the truth is that my mind was made up shortly after I'd seen the ad for the job. I suddenly remembered all of those days as a child, desperately trying to be someone my neighbors, friends, and teachers could be proud of. Instead I all too often fell from grace in one way or another. How grand it would be to triumphantly return to my hometown in the profession that I had dreamed of since fourth grade! Finally I could give them reason to be proud. I wanted the job, and for whatever reason I was fully confident that I would get it, despite the fact that as many as one hundred other applicants had also applied. I now believe that the Lord surely knew I was about to be challenged in an inevitable way, and that He wisely recognized that my coming face-to-face with my faults and weaknesses, regardless of the cost, was the only way I could become the person He wanted me to be in this life. Just as He trusted me with the remarkable witness at Cardston, I believe he trusted me to overcome the lessons I would learn in Butte as an essential part of my human life education, temporary pain and suffering notwithstanding.

Within the week, the news director at KXLF-TV, Viola Vigil, contacted me to let me know they were impressed with my résumé and tape and loved the idea that I was local. Therefore, they were offering me the job as sports director, which I accepted on the spot.

To be honest, despite the happy personal life that I led in Kalispell with my family, and occasional exciting moments at KCFW-TV there, I felt I was suffocating somewhat in such a small market. I needed to move onward, and Butte was turning into a professional dream. I fully confess, though, in time it must have become quite clear to everyone who saw me that I became a raging egomaniac from the first month there. As expected, the viewers in Anaconda couldn't have been nicer or acted more pleased to see me return. For my part, I spent many days with my news camera crew interviewing Copperheads coaches and mingling with those in town who I loved. I was more energized to be a success than at any other time in my career. Though my sports staff was small, we worked extremely hard and put in many hours covering our entire viewing area, and soon letters began pouring in about how much people appreciated the coverage and what a "fine, great sportscaster I was." While I should have humbly accepted and distributed any of those genuinely kind and sincere thoughts from the public, I instead recklessly and somewhat unwittingly allowed those sentiments to fuel a main portion of my soul that hadn't been edified: my ego. A coworker in the newsroom, Heather Jennings, once referred to the large wall behind my desk as my "ego board." At the time, I had no idea what she meant. After all, the hundreds of positive letters of great praise that I'd received and subsequently posted on that wall were something to be proud of, right? Being esteemed, approved of, and complimented was good, right? I'd worked hard my whole life to receive such accolades, so why shouldn't I proudly accept these bountiful kudos and ovations with great pride?

Oh, brother!

One thing that was certain: the ratings for our station were more than double what they ever were, and the popularity of KXLF-TV was going through the roof. To make matters better, or worse, within a year and a half I was recognized by the Greater Montana Foundation as the Montana TV Broadcaster of the Year in 1990. In those days, the TV sportscasters competed directly against all of the other news anchors, weathercasters, and reporters for that most coveted award—and I was the first and only sports guy ever to receive it against such competition. I also received a check for $1,000 and the hefty acclaim that accompanied it from across the great state. I couldn't have been more proud of myself and the achievements I had accomplished.

Oh, brother!

During that first year I clearly changed. Through all of the plaudits, cheers, and congratulations, somehow I didn't become a better person or man of God; rather, I slowly drifted into being quite the opposite.

Jeremiah 48:29

"We have heard the pride of Moab (he is exceeding proud) his loftiness, and his arrogancy, and his pride, and the hautiness of his heart."

Instead of taking my family to church at the Butte Second Ward, I began sleeping in following late night games or even staying out with those TV news team members who had gotten together for a party. I seemed to be everywhere in those days, except where I should have been. My inactivity went from weeks to months. From time to time I would drive past a church in Butte, Anaconda, or any other town and wonder what I was putting at stake as my conscience would say, "What are you doing?"

It should be noted that through it all, I never even remotely lost my testimony of the Lord even during my worst days of pride. I did find out, though, that simply having a testimony and not using it is almost worthless. Instead, it became clear to me that the more cheers I received, the worse of a person I was becoming. Not because the cheers were bad but because I was bad. Those cheers came from good people expressing genuine, positive appreciation. It was my self-consumed reactions that were bad. Slowly it was occurring to me. The recognition and notoriety that I'd tried to attain most of my life were merely attention and tributes that were fleeting and shallow. As my conceited eyes began to finally open, I began to see that much more true, personal contentment could be received via a warm smile from an elderly neighbor who I'd quietly offered a hand to rather than the cheering of 1,000 fans at the Butte Civic Center when I walked in to cover a tournament game.

Chapter 14:

Pride Precedes the Fall

THE IRONY WASN'T LOST ON ME. DURING MY
downward spiral of self-inflicted depression, the two people
key people in my life, whose lives I watched become depleted
from the same devilishly inspired anxieties growing up, were
remarkably putting their lives back together.

For a quarter of a century, Mom and Dad remained apart
physically and emotionally. Not surprisingly, it took spirituality to
close the gap. After rarely speaking or seeing each other during
those twenty-five years, I gained word from my brothers that our
parents were living in the same city in California. Bakersfield
didn't seem like a likely place my mother would ever choose
to live, but after bravely escaping her life in Montana for a new
start, she was welcomed to sunny California to live with my
brother Mike. Mike went to Bakersfield because that's where
my dad and brother Bob had wound up in pursuit of jobs in the
oil fields. So as I sat in turmoil alone in Montana, it appeared
the rest of my family was having some kind of unpredictable
family reunion of sorts after all those years.

> Revelations 2:5 "Remember therefore from
> whence thou art fallen, and repent, and do the
> first works; or else I will come unto thee quickly,
> and will remove thy candlestick out of his place,
> except thou repent."

Back in Butte, one night as I was coming home from a late-
night sports event, I came to grips with my heart, which had
been heavy for weeks as the realization of what I'd become

sank in. I was heartsick, ashamed, and embarrassed before God. When I walked into my house that evening, Nancy and our kids were fast asleep. But desperately wanting to be next to them and feel their sweet spirits, I walked to the beds of Matt, Jill, and Tyler and kneeled down in prayer to painfully confess to the Lord how I could see that I had let Him, myself, my family, and my friends down in such a self-centered way. I cried openly as I considered what I had been given just a few years before in the temple, and what I had since done with my life. I was physically sick and felt the deep wounds of worthlessness and disgust in my entire body. Praying definitely helped, and even gave me a resolve to immediately change the course of my personal and professional life to where it should have been since the first day we arrived in Butte. However, even though I strongly felt the Holy Spirit positively telling me that all could be forgiven if I would only follow through on these positive changes, as the weeks, months, and years rolled on, I simply couldn't forgive myself. Though I successfully became rededicated to being the type of active church member and example that I always wanted, and intended, to be, I foolishly allowed the adversary himself to creep into my life through feelings of guilt and depression.

In 1992 I was back to full participation in the church and even was called to be the Elder's Quorum president. I took that calling very seriously and was determined to make up for lost time by reactivating every brother in the ward I could find. I spent hours upon hours trying to contact hundreds of men who had at one time or another been active in that ward, and some good men accepted and returned to church. However, far too many would say things such as, "*You* are a Mormon?" I knew what that meant, and instead of correctly seeking the Lord through humble prayer, I allowed it to consume me in a negative way.

After all, I had been personally treated to the sweetest testimony I could ever imagine from Jesus the Christ, and how did I thank him? I began to feel the heavy weight of disgrace. I felt I wasn't worthy to represent Him, and the anguish of it soon had me on a steep downward emotional spiral. Just as I wasn't worthy to be on that pitcher's mound for the championship game, I had no business helping others find God when I was such a pathetic and ungrateful failure before the Lord. Looking back now, had I wisely adhered to the Lord's heavenly plan of repentance, I could have saved myself a great deal of very painful anguish—mentally, physically, and spiritually. After all, the Lord had already suffered infinitely for my sins. Why didn't I just humbly accept my temporary imperfections and thank Him, love Him, and trust Him after confessing to Him? How amazing that He has made it so easy for us—if we would but trust Him and return humbly.

> 2 Ne. 2:27 "The devil seeks that all men might be miserable like unto himself." Instead, I inadvertently and unwisely gave in to the influence of the adversary—not by staying away from home and family, working late-night games, or visiting company parties. This time I gave in by allowing the negative spirit of the adversary to make me feel like I had become insignificant and pointless.

> 2 Corinthians 2:11 "Lest Satan should get an advantage of us; for we are not ignorant of his devices."

Heavy depression slowly crept into my life, the results of which began to affect all aspects. I had trouble playing with the kids, talking with my wife, or even visiting a neighbor. All I wanted to do was crawl into my bed and turn off all the lights. I wondered if it was a physical disease and if it was the beginning of the end for me. Was the Lord taking my life because of what an abject failure I had become? Sadly, I got to the point where I wouldn't have blamed Him.

In the spring of 1993, my amazing wife, who had stood by my side through it all, was receiving a great honor. After several years of day and night classes, she received her college degree with high honors from Montana Tech. All of her family and friends were so proud of her. And about that time she chose to let everyone know that she was pregnant with our fourth child. It was very exciting, and we all needed that positive uplift.

Despite that, I couldn't shake my depression. I decided that late that summer I would take my family to California to visit my mom and dad for an extended two-week vacation. Surely that time would allow me to get myself together again and relax. And in fact, by the time we returned home, I did feel better, at least temporarily.

Within a few weeks I had begun a second job that I had pushed hard for. Along with continuing as the weekday TV sports anchor for KXLF, I was now going to spend my weekends as the official TV voice of the Montana State Bobcats football team. This was one of the few big assignments I had wanted to achieve but hadn't been able to, until now. Not only did it offer terrific prestige to help me build a better résumé tape to seek a better job, it provided a much-needed second paycheck. Problem was, it also required a great deal of my little free time. I had to attend all of their Saturday games, home and away, and then return to Bozeman on Sundays to tape a coaches' show to air that night across the state of Montana. As an active thirty-three-year-old man, I felt I could handle working seven days a week, but I was wrong.

> Exodus 35:2 "Six days shall work be done, but
> on the seventh day there shall be to you an holy
> day, a Sabbath of rest to the Lord."

Somewhere in the middle of that season, I began feeling sick and out of sorts. While I didn't understand it at the time, stress can affect you in many different ways. It's an insidious mental disorder that becomes physically disabling in time—often striking you the hardest in areas where you are most vulnerable at any given time. I could be sitting at my desk working on the computer and suddenly feel my heart beating quickly. Other times my vision would blur or my head would ache right before important interviews. By November, all I wanted to do was go back home, close the door in the dark, and lay there for about a month.

Depression wasn't spoken of a great deal in those days, and to even admit it seemed very embarrassing, even if I knew what it meant. So I pushed through it and simply hoped it would go away at some point. My life was miserable, and thus so was that of my young family. Ultimately, it would even affect my work. I began calling in sick for any little thing just so I could have some precious moments of quiet, in-the-dark time to myself. Nancy was extremely concerned and tried valiantly to get me to see a doctor, but I couldn't bring myself to believe I was so weak that I would need to seek help from anyone. Instead I maintained a ridiculously busy schedule as each day became more and more of a physical and mental challenge.

By this time, Nancy was nearing term with our fourth child, Randee. On December 17 she was born, and not only was I fully excited about having another adorable baby daughter, I also had a perfect excuse to take another week off work. Randee would become a child that each of us in the family would rally around. Between taking turns getting to feed her a bottle, change her diaper, or just hold her, she was a much-needed bright light of love in our lives.

Still, even that bright light couldn't illuminate the darkness of depression that was taking me over. Finally, it happened. One night in February as I was walking on the set to anchor the sportscast for KXLF-TV, as I had done most nights for the previous five years, something happened that I felt was going to end my career forever. When it came time for the sports portion of the newscast, the news anchor, Jay Kohn, leaned over to me and asked, "What's going on in sports today, Joe?"

I had spent the entire day in a severe depression. I was now shaking, having difficulty breathing, and could barely hold on to a train of thought. As Jay was asking me about sports on live television, it was like he was talking in slow motion to someone else. I had no idea what he was asking or how to answer his question. Recognizing my situation, Jay immediately called for a commercial break, and then asked me what was the matter.

I told him I simply couldn't talk. I could open my mouth, but I couldn't speak. A bit of panic began to affect the entire set because we only had two minutes to work this out before the sports segment was to come back on. No doubt, folks watching were already curious as to what the problem was with me. In an effort to snap me out of it, my good friend Jay yelled, "Knock it off, Joe! Do your job!"

I nodded my head yes and nervously awaited the end of the final commercial before the camera was back on me. When the red light came on, I did my best to simply read the teleprompter as best I could. My heart raced and I felt as though I would pass out, but I wound up finishing and quickly going back to Jay. While it was a relief to complete it, I immediately began worrying about the next night. I'd been a TV sports anchor for ten years and had never had a problem before this. *What is the matter with me?* I wondered.

The following night, as expected, I once again found that I couldn't speak a word; only this time none of Jay's promptings made a difference. By the time the camera was on me, try as I would to speak, nothing would come out. By this time, the thousands of viewers knew what I did: my career was finished. Despite pleas to stay with it and that the station was behind me 100 percent, which meant a great deal to me, I knew that I could never work there again. I was hesitant to leave my job before this since it was my only income and I had a family to care for, but at this point, I had no other choice. I came home to see Nancy very concerned. She said, "What are we going to do?"

Chapter 15:

Bakersfield to Butte

1 Corinthians 11:11 "Neither is the man without the woman in the Lord."

I OFTEN MARVEL AT HOW THE LORD HAS A PLAN set up for our lives so that even when we stumble, His plan is sufficient to pick us back up.

It had been twenty five years since I'd seen my mother and father in a loving embrace. I'd essentially forgotten the idea or even how it felt. But as my plane taxied up to the outdoor tarmac at the old Bakersfield, California, airport, I had to rub and refocus my eyes several times. Looking out the window and onto a deck that supported the family and friends awaiting their loved ones as they deboarded the plane, I saw my mother and father not only standing together for the first time since I was five, but I noted Dad's arm was around Mom that day in early March 1990. I had flown in to visit Mom. Two years earlier I moved all of Mom's things to Bakersfield, where she earned a job with Shell Oil and was able to move closer to Mike, Bob, and their families. I missed her but was very happy that she could joyously be reunited with my brothers. Knowing Dad was there, I thought it might even be possible that they could all get together from time to time. To be honest, I guess in the back of my mind was the slight chance that my mom and dad could also truly get back together again one day in some fashion. After all, they were both single. However, I always quickly gave up that thought considering how much emotional baggage they had. Surely Dad could never get over Mom's taking his family away those many years ago. And just as sure,

Mom could never take back the man who seemed to abandon her for the war. Two people who rarely ever spoke for decades could never be able to pull such a herculean task as to forgive and forget all the awful things they both no doubt remembered.

But suddenly, as enormously strange a sight as it was to see the two of them together at the airport, it dawned on me that they were, somehow, back in love. And the only possible way for that to happen successfully was through the grace of the Lord Almighty. While they both had suffered immensely during their long divorce, they both had sufficiently humbled themselves a few years earlier to seek the Lord. Against all odds, they both had fully read *The Book of Mormon* and the Holy Bible, and were consumed with the truthfulness of each. Through them, they found an abundance of humility, joy, happiness, and peace. Those two miracles would forever bless their lives… and ours. By the time Dad mustered the courage to ask Mom on their first date since the 1960s, they were both solidly active members of the Church of Jesus Christ of Latter-Day Saints. As a result, a spirit so strong and unshakeable now resided in them in a place they'd never known existed before. For his part, Dad was so strengthened that his lifelong battle with alcohol and cigarettes ended. Instead, harmony and peace dictated his life. Mom was also a changed person by that time as well. Church was her second home, and her confidence in the Lord was supreme.

In short, after all that time, I didn't recognize them… but what I did recognize was the direct hand of the Lord blessing two of His children who so needed and loved him. I have never believed in coincidence. I believe the Lord has a plan set up for each of us. That plan is designed to aid us with every breath. The better the choices we make, the more He is at liberty to bless us. Knowing that, as mortals, we would all stumble from time to time, the Lord established ways for us to return to Him. Be it through our family, friends, or our own recognition of needing Him, we each have the ability to illuminate the Light of Christ within us if we will but seek Him and keep His commandments. So it really wasn't a coincidence that in my worst professional hour, unable to speak a word on that news anchor desk, I would quickly recognize that the only place I needed and wanted to be was back home with Mom and Dad. By this time they had not only gotten remarried, they had been sealed in the temple for time and all eternity and were living happily together in a new home in California.

"Nancy, we are moving to California," I said to my dear wife, who had endured so much already. "We'll live with my Mom and Dad for a while until I get can over this." While it wasn't anything she had ever even considered before this, somehow she knew and accepted that it was probably the only way to get our lives back on track. I hadn't even asked my mom or dad if it would be okay yet, but if the Spirit had directed me to that so clearly with people so close to me, I believed it would be something they were already planning for.

Later that night I called Dad, and it seemed strangely like déjà vu. It was sixteen years earlier that I told him I would come live with him, and he was jubilant back on that day in 1977. Thankfully, and if possible, he seemed every bit as pleased with this call. "Having You, Nancy, and the kids stay with us will be a great joy and pleasure. You can arrive anytime and stay as long as you possibly can or want to," was his heroic response.

Those words were precisely the ones I wanted and needed to hear. Not only would we be able to once again spend time together, it could also help replace those lost childhood years. We all knew that, and all looked forward to it. Additionally, my parents would also have a unique opportunity to be with their four grandchildren and dear daughter-in-law. Mom made it clear that she too was equally thrilled. Starting that night, the two of them immediately began making all arrangements needed to have a full family of six move in with them. My aching heart needed this.

From the first day we arrived in early May 1994, all of our lives were filled with the happiness and joy of being one great big family. Rarely in life do we receive "do-overs," and we were all determined to make the most of this one. Dad had huge orange and lemon trees in his backyard, along with a large garden he said our kids could raid anytime they liked. When the kids were at school, I would often go out in their large, enclosed backyard and sit facing the sun. I prayed, meditated, and eventually found I could defeat the depressions that ravaged me.

93

We wound up spending nearly four months with them in Bakersfield. Through his own painful experiences, Dad knew firsthand what depression was, and of the few ways to overcome it. Mom was well versed in it too. Together they provided such a harmonious home life that by the early summer I was back to myself and ready to move on in a grand way. I'll never forget the love and dedication to each of us that my parents showed. How could I?

I had made arrangements to move my family to Utah, where I felt strongly prompted to take classes at Weber State University in Ogden while I began a search for full-time work. A bit strange, considering I had no idea where Weber County was.

> Psalms 1 19:12 "Blessed art thou, O Lord: teach me thy statues."

I was temporarily perplexed the day we arrived in Ogden, given my full understanding through the Holy Ghost that the Lord had intended for us to relocate there.

Fully expecting to immediately find a great, affordable home to move into that day, I would receive another lesson in patience. In fact, after arriving early in the morning that day in mid-June, I immediately began pursuing all avenues that would presumably lead to our new housing. In fact, I spent about eight hours searching through newspaper listings of all types and other advertisements, only to find nothing at all. We then wound up driving for a couple hours searching for HOUSE FOR RENT signs, and could find none. By dinnertime that night, I admit to becoming discouraged. I'm sure my family was too, although I did my best to put on a brave face by telling them, "Good things come to those who wait… and I was already told we would find a place here today."

So confident was I that I'd have a place lined up earlier in the day, I had also planned to drive another six hours to Anaconda and stay at Nancy's mother's home that night. Partially as a way to help us out financially, Joan had offered me a large house-painting job, and I was eager to begin right away. But now, with an unexpected possibility of having to stay in Utah for another day or longer, I began wondering if I would have to spend time in a hotel or put out for other expenses during my search for a place to live.

> 1 Thessalonians 1:3 "Remembering without ceasing your work of faith, and labour of love, and patience of hope in our Lord Jesus Christ, in the sight of God and our Father."

I had been so sure about this. In fact, I'd boldly proclaimed before leaving California that morning to Nancy and the kids that I was strongly assured through the Holy Ghost that we'd secure housing that day. I also saw that they'd faithfully trusted and believed me. Yet there I was aimlessly driving the Ogden city streets wondering what had happened. As I drove the family to a fast food restaurant on Harrison Avenue, I left them to order while I retreated to the men's room to wash and ponder. I then stepped out to a quiet area on the grounds and offered up a heartfelt prayer to the Lord. "Father in Heaven, I am feeling confused. I *know* that thou wanted me to come this day, and I have done the things I felt prompted to do. I continue to have faith at this late hour of the day. Please bless me and my family."

> Psalms 61:1 "Hear my cry, O God; attend unto my prayer."

On my way back out to our table, I noticed a lady gleefully chatting with Nancy. I wondered hopefully, *Is this a miracle of some sort?* Sure enough, Nancy informed me that since this kindly woman had just moved into a new house, she asked Nancy if we were interested in her old home. I wanted to shout out "Hallelujah!" Another lesson learned.

With that, we finished our meal and I decided to drive straight up to Anaconda that night. I was eager to begin working the job that Joan had lined up, and besides, we didn't have money for a hotel.

In the very city I had been working in as a sportscaster the past five years, Joan owned a house and had hired me to handle the job of scraping and repainting it. It was actually the home she had grown up in as an only child, so I knew it also

95

meant a great deal to her. As a TV broadcaster, few were the times when I actually had to get down and dirty in my work. And I have to admit even I didn't know what I was in for. Scraping old paint off an old home is not easy work. As drops of sweat poured off my face, I started to wonder if I was really up to it. Matt and Jill would take some shifts with me during several of the days, and those moments were priceless to me. Not once did either of them ever complain to me. My love and appreciation for them couldn't have been greater.

I intended for this job to last at least a week, but some ten days later I was still struggling to complete it. While most of the laborious scraping was completed, the home's shingles provided many challenging issues for a proper painting. One memorable day, as I was at the home by myself, I noticed a patch of old paint on the upper front deck of the house. I put down my brush and lined up my ladder in an effort to reach it before painting. Crawling carelessly up a shaky ladder, knowing that I'd previously fallen a time or two on other occasions in front of my startled kids, I slowly carried the scraper in one hand and the can of paint in the other. That obviously left no hand to secure on the ladder. By the time I was up there around fifteen feet, I lost my balance. The result of which sent me flailing downward with all my gear splashing onto me as I hit the grass.

While I felt blessed not to have been seriously injured physically, I was about to learn a great lesson in humility. Those five years I'd spent working as a sportscaster in the area were far from noteworthy examples of humbleness. In fact, even though I'd returned to church and believed I was doing a decent job representing all that I believed it, my arrogance was often palpable. I'm embarrassed to this day at the degree of conceit and arrogance I carried around with me. Often my wife would attempt to bring me back down to earth, but in time I would drift back into egotism. Part of it came with the job, I suppose. But the great majority of it came from my own unexorcised pretension and foolish pride. Looking back, I wonder if it was the product of feeling others considered me worthless as a young child, all while believing there was something more special in me that I hadn't presented yet to them. To that point, I

96

had erroneously incorrectly believed that it was my fascinating ability to broadcast that made me special.

Oh, brother!

Around that same time, LDS president Ezra Taft Benson had given an important conference talk titled, "Beware of Pride." Had I been listening to him and not off working or playing, I could have saved myself a great deal of heartache.

As I lay on the ground, shaken from the harrowing fall off the ladder and covered with paint and mud, it happened. Two young men roughly in their mid-twenties came walking by on the front sidewalk. In my disgraceful shame, I hid my face in my work gloves, but it was too late. They both walked up to the fence and stared. I knew what they were thinking: *Could this be him? The once puffed-up and self-important former KXLF-TV sportscaster who left a few months back?*

"You're Joe Wren!" one shouted in amusement, looking at the ignominious position I was now. "Ha ha ha! Man, you sure aren't anything now, are ya?" he laughed as they walked off.

If anyone had ever wondered at that point if I'd received all the humbling I had coming to me, they could relax. As I watched them walk off, jubilant in my fall, it became very obvious how correct they were. My fall was tremendous, and as I lay there I felt my shame was great. I guess I'd been fooling myself all those years, because I was nothing at all. I felt so small and worthless that I couldn't even stand. I wasn't even worth crying over to myself. *It's over*, I thought.

Dichotomy being what it is, I could easily witness the amazing thing that happened to me then. There I was in what had to be the worst, most humiliating and alienated point in my life, starting to laugh. I laughed hard and I laughed out loud. Joy roared back into my heart and soul as I did so. In the most wonderfully uplifting way, the Holy Spirit came into my life and said, "Finally!" In other words, finally I could see that the worth of souls has nothing to do with great fame, fortune, or how successful you are in business. Joy came through giving those things up and loving and caring for others more than yourself. It was the only way I could have learned such a supremely important lesson.

97

Proverbs 22:4 "By humility and the fear of the Lord are riches, and honour, and life." While I'm far from perfect and far from being as humble as I should be all the time, I learned a great and valuable lesson that day. It was one that would have made my life much better if I'd only learned it earlier, but I'll be forever grateful to the clear and obvious way the Lord chose to present it to me that day.

Chapter 16:

The Day I Died

Job 24:17 "For the morning is to them even as
the shadow of death; If one know them, they are
in the terrors of the shadow of death."

THE SUMMER OF 2016 WAS SO EXCITING FOR
Nancy and me. Almost daily we would discuss our awesome vacation plans schedule for Labor Day weekend. Not
only were we going to fly into Phoenix to see the opening football game of the major college season, but we'd also chosen to
splurge a bit by reserving a room at a classy hotel across the
street from the NFL stadium where the game would be played.
As we studied our itinerary, we were also excited at the idea
of attending many of the fun activities scheduled around the
game and the area of Glendale. Over the years, we'd become
great fans of Brigham Young University football and tried to
catch at least one away game during the past few seasons. In
2015 we saw a thrilling battle at the Rose Bowl in Pasadena
as BYU met UCLA.

This time, on a professional field that would be broadcast on national television, BYU would be playing the Pac-12
Arizona Wildcats.

Every few nights that summer we'd pull out our game plan of
anticipated events for that weekend and review. I even worked
a shift on local sports radio and discussed why I thought BYU
would upset their Pac-12 opponent that day. The Cougars had
a new coach, Kilani Sitaki, who was loved. He had a great way
of bringing love to his players, coaches, and us fans. Everything

99

was set for what we were confident would be an exciting and emotional weekend. And was it ever…

As the days led up to our Friday, September 2, flight to Arizona, we had many details to line up. For one thing, our son Tyler had just purchased a beautiful new home in Fruit Heights, Utah, for his lovely wife and identical twin daughters, Eden and Gracie May. A few nights before leaving, we joined all of our other children and grandchildren for a housewarming night to tour Tyler's new residence. By that time we had eleven grandchildren to go with our four kids. Matt was thirty-six and joined by his darling wife, Michelle, and their three terrific children, Lauren, Reese, and Charlie. Our oldest daughter, Jill, was thirty-four, married to a fine man named Dave, and had four children: Ally, Emily, Daniel, and Katherine. Our youngest daughter, Randee, was twenty-three, had married an amazing young man named Deven, and together they had two sweet daughters in Ella and Indie.

Honestly, the only downfall leading up to that weekend trip was the idea of having to leave behind these family members whom we adored so much. Emotionally and spiritually we were flying high already. We recognized how blessed we were with family and friends in abundance.

However, physically I was having a few problems that I'd kept to myself that spring and summer. For several years I had dealt with some minor pains in my chest, back, and arms. The pain rotated and seemed to go away after my daily workouts. I had been very active in physical activities almost daily for the past thirty years, including long jogs and climbing steep mountains. About seven years earlier, when I first began feeling the pain in my left arm when I exerted myself in exercise, I decided to ask my doctor to schedule an appointment to have a stress test done at the hospital. He almost didn't want to do it, considering what great shape I was in and how busy the hospitals were with other patients who were in need. But eventually I was penciled in and able to be hooked up with numerous monitors while I jogged on the treadmill at high speeds to get my heart rate as high as they could safely take it before checking all my heart points. Almost immediately I was told that everything was fine, which gave me the relief I needed to continue on my rigorous schedule of daily athletics.

Back in the summer of 2014, I pushed the endurance envelope a little by taking Randee and Tyler to beautiful Mt. Haggin in southwest Montana. It is one of the tallest peaks in the state at nearly 12,000 feet, and for those who are fortunate enough to make it to the peak, it offers a spectacular view for a hundred miles in each direction. As we began our ascent to the top, just a few miles into the hike, I felt that familiar tightness in my left arm. I remember thinking to myself, *Oh, Lord, please allow me to make this hike without suffering a heart attack!* On the surface, it almost seemed silly for me to even ask that, given the stress test results and my otherwise great health, but for some reason I felt that calling upon my Father in heaven was the right thing to do. Ultimately, after taking a wrong turn or two on the hike, we wound up covering nearly twenty-four miles of rugged terrain that day. I look back now and can plainly see the Lord's hand in assuring through rich blessings that nothing dreadful would happen to me on such an arduous hike, given the declining health position I was already unknowingly in. The three of us, exhausted but jubilant over what we had done, returned to town early that evening and were greeted at the gate by Dad. His glowing face exuded great pride at the sight of us three dusty and worn-out campers.

Tyler was even more proud that night as we gathered in and around his brand-new home. He had been an extremely bright and successful young man almost since birth. From his scholastic abilities to his national championships in athletics, Tyler has always been seen as one who sets and achieves the highest standards and goals. How difficult it was that day back in 2006 when we dropped him off at the Missionary Training Center to say good-bye for two years. But how much joy it gave us to hear word that on the very first day of his Buffalo, New York, assignment, his mission president had taken him to the Sacred Grove. Many was the night the past few years before his leaving that I would open his bedroom door to say good night, only to see him studying the scriptures quietly alone. By the time he'd left, he knew virtually every scripture I could ask him about. He also did it precisely as the Lord would have him: humbly and honestly.

The only problem I had that final night of the family touring Tyler and Heather's new home was a growing uneasiness about my health. Over the couple years before that night, my pains had begun to increase in my back and chest. Things got so bad that six months before, as I practiced for my first pickleball tournament coming up over Memorial Day, I would have to lay down on the court several times a match until my pains subsided. I contacted my doctor a few times to tell him, but I did so in a relaxed way. I figured I was fine and didn't want to take him away from his patients with real issues. I'd even sent him a text a time or two suggesting that I return to the hospital for further checkups. He agreed to that and told me he would set it up if I so chose. But I foolishly chalked up my grave condition to stress or a pulled muscle. Putting off such pains and a trip to the emergency room, as I've since learned and counseled thousands others, is a very poor idea.

Despite all deepening and increased consistency of my pain, I pushed on. We even came back to win a medal at the pickleball tournament we'd prepared for, even though I was experiencing a good deal of pain throughout. Along with that excruciating pain, and likely as a result of it, I recall my personality changing somewhat. Conversations and attitudes toward my children, friends, and even my darling wife, Nancy, seemed to be less cheerful and more impatient. In the back of my mind those final years, and especially that last summer, I was becoming increasingly alarmed at what was happening, despite not understanding it all. The fact that my condition became worse very gradually made things even worse. I tried taking more time off work, relaxing more, and eating better. Temporarily those things would help, but my body was beginning to scream at me about the poor shape it was in.

As we finished visiting and touring Tyler's house that evening before our scheduled Arizona trip, I suddenly began feeling faint and a little shaky. Thinking it was simply from being overtired at not having slept well for a few weeks, I walked off alone for a lengthy period of time to try and recover. I prayed that I would be taken care of in whatever way was needed. Weeks later, Randee's mother-in-law, Cheri, would admit to me that when she saw me that day she was concerned. She said my face looked gray and gaunt. The excitement of our upcoming trip, however, kept me pumped up and motivated.

Finally, that fateful day of September 2 arrived. It was a particularly early Friday morning for me, given I slept poorly and was up by 5:30 AM. Given the hour, I decided to make the most of my early rise by going in to work for an hour or so to make sure all details were taken care of. Afterward, since I had my shorts and tennis shoes in the car anyway, I chose to drive to Monroe Park in Ogden to play an hour or so of pickleball with my friends. It was a decision that ultimately cost me my life, as well as returned it.

It was a warm, sunny morning that already saw ten or more players gathered on the courts. I acknowledged the many friends who were there, including Rusty Jensen and Bob McFarland. Bob was the owner of his own Ford dealership in Brigham City, but you'd never know of his extended professional successes because he was such a thoughtful and uplifting person. Rusty was a man who had become a close friend through our almost daily games of pickleball. President Jensen had recently been called to serve in the Stake Presidency of the Ogden East Stake. A strong man of God who could always be counted on.

Though they all came to greet me and say hi, I wasn't in any mood for discussion. In fact, I didn't even feel like playing that day. My pains were present, and my energy was almost nonexistent. In spite of this, or perhaps because of it, I decided some exercise might do me some good, so I approached the court and started what would be a final competitive doubles match. Such was my frame of mind that I don't even remember whom I was playing with or against.

All my mind could focus on was the increasingly unusual feelings of discomfort in my chest, arms, and back. I do know that we'd fallen behind by five points and were on the verge of defeat. Being most competitive, and despite the extremely precariously situation of dangerous health I was unknowingly in, I decided we were *not* going to lose that match. I then mustered up every last bit of energy that I had, and vigorously attacked every successful shot I could think of.

My final volley was a gorgeous winner up the baseline. Oh, how many times I've since thought of how correct PGA star Jack Nicklaus was when he told me, "Winning a game should never be overemphasized because it can never compare to the truly important things in life!"

As we performed our customary post-match handshake at the net for congratulations, my mind couldn't be further away from the win.

"Great game, Joe. You did it!" my partner said to me as I began slipping into a cloudy, full-on daze, likely typical of one who is about to die. Mechanically I forced myself to walk off the court. Four or five steps was enough to get me past the gate and onto the sidewalk that separated the courts.

At that point, it became abundantly clear to me my life was now fully in the hands from heaven.

"Yell out, 9-1-1!" was the utterly unmistakable shout I heard. Yet miraculously it hadn't come from any earthly being. This heartfelt and solemn warning came as a direct gift from the Lord Almighty through the Holy Ghost. No earthly being would have or could have gained my absolute and immediate attention, even as I precariously hovered in such a cadaverous condition. In fact, though dying, my body felt consumed by the Holy Spirit, making it so undeniably clear, even in those final seconds before death, that I heard, listened, and obeyed.

"Call 9-1-1!" were my final words, projected just one second after receiving that heaven-sent prompting. From there, I was finished. I vaguely remember my knees buckling, but in the very short time it took for me to fall to the ground, I was fully unconscious.

Prior to this moment, I had no idea who Kent Smedley was. In fact, the first time I recall meeting him was by chance— seven months later. He later wrote me with this firsthand witness of what happened.

"I was playing pickleball in Ogden at the Monroe Parks court with three friends," wrote Smedley. As I went to serve the ball, I noticed that the game which was being played on the court next to ours had come to an immediate and abrupt halt. I also saw players huddled around what appeared to be a man laying on the ground. We quickly threw down our paddles and ran to see if our help could be offered. What we witnessed when we arrived was two men giving frantic CPR to their lifeless friend.

"To be honest, it seemed as though the efforts were futile as the unresponsive man was motionless for five full minutes. My friend and I made eye contact and were moved to turn away from the group and openly pray. As we returned, the man who we found to be Joe Wren was just taking his first breath! From there, we began seeing joyous signs of hope as he would open his eyes briefly before closing them again.

"Each time he would struggle to reopen his eyes, a loud chorus of us would yell out, 'Joe, you can do this!' as though we were cheering for a sports hero at a football game."

Chapter 17:

John 11:25 "I am the resurrection, and the life: he that believeth in me, though he were dead, yet shall he live."

THROUGHOUT MY LIFE I'D EXPERIENCED VARIOUS degrees of excruciating pain and severe fright, but I can honestly say that I hadn't ever felt anything as mortally acute as I did an hour or so later as I was returned to earthly consciousness. Initially, with my eyes still closed, I heard anxious voices screaming medical instructions and yelling for people to clear out of the way. It was an out-of-body experience that had me as confused as I was frightened. As I struggled mentally to picture in my mind what was happening, I soon realized that these were emergency medical teams desperately attempting to save some poor soul in a clearly critical and life-threatening situation. I became very concerned for whomever it was struggling so close to death.

Then it came to me.

Ironically similar to my favorite Christmas story *A Christmas Carol*, which notes the moment Ebenezer Scrooge recognized it was his own tombstone that the Ghost of Christmas Future was pointing to, I frightfully realized I was the man who was at death's doorstep. The only way for me to describe that feeling is to say to consider your very worst nightmare that you awoke from, and multiply it by one hundred or more.

By that time, many of my closest family members had been notified and one by one were ascending to the emergency entrance of McKay Dee Hospital in Ogden. Early on they were notified only that my condition was dire enough that each of them needed to be there, perhaps just to see me one more time.

My eyes barely open and my mind still attempting to understand what was going on, I meekly peeked out in the direction of familiar sounds and saw Matt, Tyler, my younger brother Troy, and my dear wife, Nancy, staring back at me with exceeding concern on their faces. They had been given permission to stand by and watch me pass as the EMT team rushed my rolling bed from the ambulance and toward the medical emergency room to determine what, if anything, could be done to save my life.

But then, in the most intense of moments, my entire mental, spiritual, and even physical faculties changed almost immediately. "Many, many dear souls are praying for you." That was the next clear voice I heard. Only, again, it wasn't coming from a friend, wife, or doctor; it was coming from the Holy Ghost Himself.

My first thought upon hearing such a still, small but vocally clear and unmistakable voice was, *Very cool... but what are they praying for?* Regardless, I was so moved that I began praying with them. At the time, I hadn't any idea what was wrong with me, nor did I know how so many people would even be aware of the dreadful situation I was in. Only later would I learn that at that very moment, many hundreds of friends and family members had already been notified by phone, text, emails, and even Facebook, including via a special page I had begun myself for the thousands of my hometown friends I had in Montana called "Anaconda—Always." As I read their heartwarming thoughts and prayers in the weeks to follow, my heart was filled and filled again with joy in Christ, knowing that His love had inspired such goodness and positive light for so many.

That light erupted in me as I lay there, even as I heard doctors' voices describing their desperate efforts to save my life. The light I speak of was the burning ember of the Holy Ghost. Physically, it was dark in that emergency operating room, but spiritually my mind was now intensely illuminated by the power of the Holy Ghost, and I knew I was not alone. In words that are not nearly suitable to describe it all, I will say that I was consumed with the spiritual presence of God the Father and Jesus Christ. How it was that they would appear to me, far from perfect and seemingly of little consequence considering the state of the world, personally astounded me, but it was so real that I wholeheartedly accepted their love and accompaniment.

Other than the eight words the Holy Ghost clearly spoke to me, no other actual "words" were expressed, but I can assure all that visitations like that require very few words.

All this joy and unspeakable love from on high, even as I lay in a near-terminal state hovering in and out of death. My doctors would later confirm that it had been their experience that the chances of anyone actually living through the morning I was struggling through were less than 5 percent.

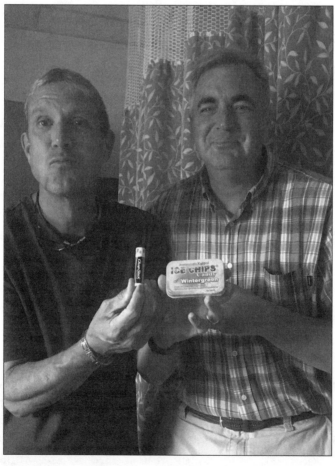

The two men who rushed to my side to perform life-saving CPR at Monroe Park, Rusty Jensen (right) and Bob McFarland, visiting me at McKay Dee Hospital prior to my open heart surgery.

"Make no mistake; he had died!" noted Eric Lindley, the McKay Dee Hospital emergency doctor in charge of my care that morning.

I would later learn that immediately after I'd collapsed on the court, Rusty and Bob began the necessary and life-saving actions of cardiopulmonary resuscitation. Inspired by the Lord, Rusty took charge. Only recently had he agreed to take classes on CPR, which his sister taught at local hospitals and had long invited him to take. As Bob began to clear my throat and initiate mouth-to-mouth resuscitation, a pair of senior missionaries who had been there for some fellowshipping and exercise began praying aloud beside me.

While I had no knowledge of where they were, what they were doing at the time, or how they were finding out about the shocking news of my massive heart attack, virtually my entire family would hear about my desperate predicament before I did.

"I was in the living room of my sister's house in Colorado when I got the phone call," Noted my youngest daughter, Randee, then twenty-two years old. "My call was coming from my brother-in-law, Dave. We didn't talk much on the phone, so this was strange. I quickly answered, having a gut feeling something was wrong. 'Hello,' I said. 'Randee, its Dave. Have you talked to anyone?', he asked. 'No, what's going on?' I asked, with a sick feeling inside. 'Your dad had a heart attack.' My mind quickly raced back to the week before when we were playing pickleball at my brother Matt's house. Matt and I were playing against Dad, and he would stop periodically to stretch his back as if he were in pain. The phone call from Dave was a shock, but it was almost as if I knew it was coming from the signs I saw before. As I got off the phone, I quickly knelt down and said a prayer in the quiet home. As I opened my eyes, I felt the words come into my mind, 'All will be well.' I wasn't completely sure at that moment what that meant, but I felt such peace that I knew no matter the outcome, God had a plan. Though I felt peace, it was a frightening feeling being miles away from your father while not knowing whether I'd see him or talk with him again in this life. That was the hardest part—being so far away and feeling so helpless.

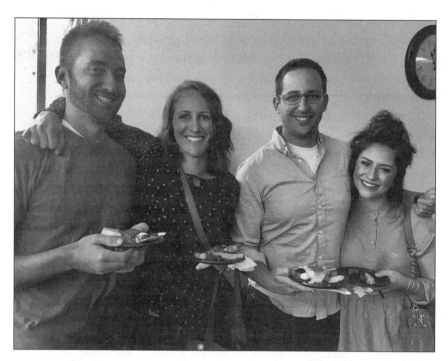

My four kids, Tyler, Jill, Matt and Randee optimistically awaiting positive word while I was in quadruple bi-pass surgery at McKay-Dee Hospital.

"After my sister and I ran around the house like madwomen packing up the family to drive back to Utah, we reminisced about all the memories we had with our dad. We were truly blessed with a father who spent so much time with us. We had so many memories, it kept us occupied during the eight-hour drive back home. Walking in and seeing my dad alive and talking in the hospital room was such a tender mercy I will be forever grateful to God for."

Around the same time that Randee and Jill heard of my situation while in Colorado, my sons Matt and twenty-nine-year-old Tyler were also receiving the word. Ironically Tyler, a former U.S. National Singles Open Division National Champion, was playing in a pickleball tournament in Brigham City. Meanwhile, Matt recalled he was at work when he heard. "On September 2, 2016, we experienced a tragedy as well as a major miracle," recalled Matt. "Some people know him as Happy Joe, his grandkids know him as Papa Joe, but as kids we knew him simply as our kind and loving dad, who would give anything in the whole world for us. That morning I was at an appointment with one of my customers when I received two text messages from my little brother and a phone call from my mom. I knew that it must be urgent, so I took a quick phone call from Mom and she explained that Dad had collapsed while playing pickleball. She didn't know the extent of the situation but was heading to the hospital. A few minutes later I spoke with my little brother, Tyler, who had a bit more information and explained that my dad had actually suffered a major heart attack and needed to be resuscitated by CPR from some friends who had been playing pickleball with him until the paramedics arrived. It was at that moment that the reality of the situation sank in and I faced the reality that I may never see my dad again.

"I hadn't experienced too many tragic events in my life, so this phone call and my drive home will be one of those events that will stay with me throughout my life. Immediately my heart and mind turned to the only thing that I felt I could do. I prayed to Heavenly Father almost the entire drive home. I prayed that Dad would be okay and that we would have a chance to be with him again. As I prayed, I somehow felt confident that Dad was going to be okay, but when we made it to the hospital and the doctor explained the situation, it became very clear how miraculous it was for Dad to have survived even to this point. I experienced a roller coaster of emotions that morning. I felt sadness and distress for my dad, complete heartache for my mom, all while feeling overwhelmingly indebtedness to Dad's friends and medical professionals who had helped save his life. Most important, I was eternally grateful to Heavenly Father for extending Dad's life, giving me the opportunity to share more experiences with him.

"Once my dad was stabilized, we were allowed a few brief moments to share with him. It was during that time that we were able to bestow upon him a priesthood blessing. I'll never forget crowding in a small ICU recovery room (that was only big enough for two people) with my brother Tyler, Uncle Troy, and Mom. Revelation flowed abundantly as we placed our hands gently on Dad's head. He was promised many special blessings, one of which was that he would be able to share this experience with others and relate the divinity of Heavenly Father's plan of happiness as well as the living Savior of the world. There was no doubt in my mind that Papa Joe would heal in time and would live to bear his witness of what really matters most. It has been said that 'Man's extremity is God's opportunity,' and that is exactly how I felt on September 2, 2016."

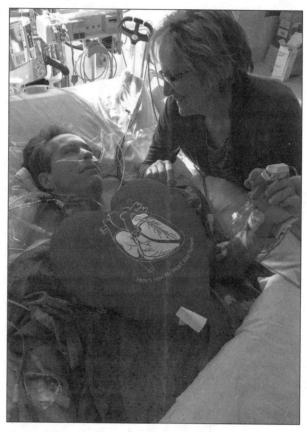

Nancy by my side hours after my quadruple bi-pass open heart surgery at McKay Dee Hospital.

"For me," recalled my oldest daughter, Jill, "the main things that stand out when thinking about that time are:

1. Family ties are meant to be forever, and there is no doubt about it. The eight-hour drive to Utah seemed endless and at times was filled with many questions. The first one being, 'Is Dad's heart going to be strong enough for us to see him when we arrive?' We didn't know if he would be alive when we got

there. But every time I felt nervous and questioned how this could turn out positively, the thought, 'No matter what happens, you will always be together' ran though my mind and calmed me from head to toe. I also was reminded many times that we are strangers on the earth; this world is not our final destination. With confidence in those truths, I realized we could relax and not worry about death.

2. The power of prayer offers confidence and peace. Not long after hearing the news and the severity of Dad's condition, I felt the Spirit say, 'Did you remember to pray?' Immediately I got on my knees and I noticed that my prayer was being heard. Out of all the prayers I offered in my life, this was something I'd never actually felt before. It was as if angels were giving my words special treatment and my message was being expedited. This experience helped me to feel greater confidence in the knowledge that our prayers are recognized and delivered. Whether they are our consistent daily prayers, our prayers in our hearts, or those of a pleading nature, we are heard, we are loved, and we are strengthened. When we gain testimony of this important power, peace comes. It's really pretty neat.

3. All things will give us experience. As difficult as it was to watch my dad struggle through anxiety and anticipation before the surgery, the emotional pain of recovery, or the later physical discomforts of his efforts to restrengthen his heart and body, I realized that this was all for a purpose. Clearly life can throw curve balls at unexpected times, but if instead we can embrace these experiences as growing opportunities, we will recover with greater gusto and desire to move forward with strength and faith. Once, many years ago, I felt the Spirit teach me that the quicker I search to learn why I'm being taught a lesson, the sooner the struggle seems less daunting and more manageable. Difficult experiences help me to be ever so grateful that the Savior desired to feel what we feel so that we may draw closer to Him. He has felt what we feel. It's so nice to have an empathetic friend, isn't it?'

Tyler has also been a soul who has sought the Lord throughout his life. He has a special gift of success in almost everything he sets out to do. Blessed with a brilliant mind that often resembles a photographic memory, oftentimes friends ask how he can be so perfect at almost everything, but what they don't always know is the price he's paid for such abilities. He has a special connection with the Lord but also is subject to reconciling that spirit with a mind that demands perfection in ways I don't always understand. Yet he goes about his way daily, living the way the Lord wants him to and being a bright light before us all.

"The Tournament of Champions is the largest money tournament in pickleball," Tyler explained when recalling that fateful day in September. "Players from all over the country travel to the small town of Brigham City, Utah, to compete for over $50,000 in prize money. I had been training all year in preparation against the best in the country. I was in the middle of my first match of the day when I heard my phone ringing. I forgot to put it on silent! After the point, I called a timeout and ran over to turn it off. I won my first match and was looking forward to the next. I walked over to look and my phone and noticed multiple missed calls and text messages, almost all of which were coming from a friend, Rusty Jensen. I listened to one of the voice mails and heard Rusty's voice—'Hello? Tyler, are you there? Keep breathing, Joe, stay with me. Tyler, are you there? Can you hear me?' Then he hung up. I had a text from him saying, 'Tyler, it's Rusty. Call me immediately. It's an emergency.'

"My heart started racing. I called him right away, and he answered and told me my dad had collapsed playing pickleball. He wasn't doing well, and the ambulance had just come to take him away. He was pretty shaken up, and I had lots going through my mind, so I asked if my mom knew yet, and he said he didn't have her number. I told him I needed to call her and hung up. I spoke with my mom, and she had heard he had fainted at the courts. I asked if I should drop out and come down, but she said he was probably okay and maybe just got dehydrated or something. She was going to go to the hospital to check on him and said she'd call if she heard anything but not to worry. Just then I got called to my next match. After my second round I checked my phone and saw more missed calls. I called my mom, and she gave me the bad news. It was a lot more serious than we had thought. He had a massive heart attack and was fighting to stay alive. He'd be going in for surgery soon. I ran to the tournament desk to inform them I'd have to drop out. It was about a thirty-minute drive to Ogden, but it seemed to last hours.

"My anxiety was going crazy, and I couldn't control my racing heart. I felt dizzy and was nervous I might pass out driving down the highway. I remember praying the whole way but to no avail. Then all of a sudden, as I was waiting at a red light on 40th and Washington, I felt an overwhelming feeling of comfort and a voice said, 'Everything will be okay.' I wasn't sure if that referred to my dad's health or that everything would eventually work out, but I didn't care. I felt at peace. I soon arrived at the hospital and met my family. Just then, they wheeled my dad out on a stretcher to briefly say hi. We asked if we could provide a priesthood blessing, and the nurse said that would be more help than anything she could do. I performed the anointing and my brother gave the blessing. Immediately I had a second assurance that not only would everything eventually work out but that my dad would make a full recovery. I knew that hundreds of prayers were being offered on behalf of my dad, myself, and the rest of my family, and I received a witness then that God was listening and cared. I'm forever grateful for the power of prayer, priesthood, and friendship that provided much-needed comfort during a tumultuous time."

Some twenty years earlier, my dad had suffered a mild heart attack of his own after moving to the Orem, Utah, area in 1996. Despite that health setback, he and my mom's renewed marriage continued to be blessed, and they were living happily and harmoniously, even taking eighteen months out of their time to serve a church mission to Paris, France. After returning home, they lived in Bakersfield for several years before returning to Anaconda to build a home. My older brother Mike, who had long since longed to spend quality time with his parents, was able to build a home large enough for himself, Mom and Dad, and his wife, Sharon, in a beautiful area west of town.

All was going well there for the first four months after moving in, until that day in September when my parents heard their son was close to death in an Ogden Hospital.

"My husband, Bob, and I were going about our usual morning activities that otherwise sunny September morning," Mom recalled. "Suddenly, our daughter-in-law Sharon entered our room and asked me where Bob was. I replied he was out-side working, and she said, 'Please get him in here right away.' Well, I knew something was wrong then, and a terrible feeling of dread came over me. When we were gathered together, Sharon gave us the unbelievable news that our son Joe had collapsed on a pickleball court in Utah and that he had been given CPR for a lengthy period of time and was being trans-ferred to the hospital via emergency vehicle! What? We were both astounded! Could this be possible? Our son Joe had always taken such good care of himself by exercising daily, playing strenuous games with his two sons, Matt and Tyler, and more. Upon hearing this news we immediately had a heartfelt prayer, grabbed a suitcase, threw in it everything we thought we might need for an indefinite period of time, jumped in the car, and were on our way to Utah in less than an hour. That drive was a nightmare of fear and hope, tears and prayer.

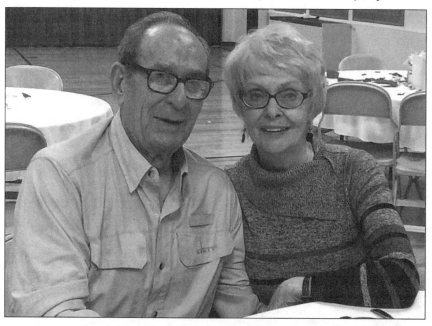

Mom and dad in 2017

"Bob, Joe's Dad, upon hearing the news immediately said, 'We're going right now!' His first thought was getting to Joe as fast as we possibly could, and he drove the eight-hour trip with that in mind! He recalls the terrible fear and dread, of feelings of heaviness in his chest, of disbelief, and recalling his deep love for Joe and how important he was to his happiness and to all of our happiness in this life. What a terrible shock it was to receive this scary news! It was unbelievable, and yet it had actually happened, and we knew it! It was a heart-wrenching trip, not knowing how Joe was and what might be the dreadful end to this nightmare. However, we prayed all the way and held out hope that Heavenly Father would spare Joe's life.

"When Dad and I finally arrived at the hospital, we found to our great relief that Joe was lying in his bed talking with his company gathered around him, and even laughing. It wasn't long before all his beloved Utah grandchildren were piled on the hospital bed with him receiving his love and good humor. We shook our heads in disbelief, not realizing yet that during his time of unconsciousness Joe had been blessed with such an amazing experience that now he was not even afraid of what had happened or what could actually happen! He told us not to worry and that he had no fear of death, and we could tell he wasn't only trying to comfort us but that he really meant it.

"For the next few days, while the physicians were delaying the necessary surgery until Joe's poor heart had time to heal some from the damage the attack had done, Joe behaved almost as if the terrible, life-threatening heart attack had not even happened. How could he be cheerful after coming so terribly close to dying? Soon his excellent physician, who was also Joe's stake president, stood stately in the hospital room with most of Joe's family around him and informed us of the procedure that would be necessary to keep Joe alive. We knew Joe had a great surgeon whom he trusted, and that helped calm our fears. None of us will forget the heart-wrenching farewells as we left his room on the eve of his heart operation.

"The waiting room at the hospital was a mighty quiet and somber place for hours while we waited and prayed for the results of the surgery. Finally one of the doctors came into the waiting room and announced the great news that the surgery

117

was over and had gone very well. Immediately, we all collapsed to our knees in tears and had a grateful family prayer to Heavenly Father and Jesus Christ for saving Joe. Even Nancy, who had tried so hard to be strong around all of us and the children, finally had to cave in and cry her heart out with relief and gratitude. I will never forget that beautiful scene.

"It wasn't until after the quadruple bypass that Joe finally showed the life-threatening ordeal he had been through, with tubes running everywhere and a very sick countenance. We were so very grateful, though, for there having been a way for him to be healed and hopefully have a normal life again. Joe's life has been renewed in such a marvelous way that he and none of us will ever be quite the same. He had always brought laughter and good cheer to every group he was in, and now to that has been added a new and even stronger testimony of our Lord and Savior, Jesus Christ, and His power to love and save lives."

"Along with the sweet presence of a glorious family, my still-beating heart would also be filled that week by the surprising and heartfelt efforts of both Mike Strizich and Tom Oberweiser, who overcome personal obstacles to remarkably be at my hospital bedside. Each traveled many miles by car and plane to see me for what was nearly the last time. My heart swelled as I caught glimpses of both of them flying past my hospital door desperately searching for the room I was in. Tracy, being sickly himself, was unable to be there—but I haven't any doubts that he would have if at all possible. We are three very different, but very much alike brothers, and sons of God. I love them, just as I love all of my dear family and friends from the town my life began in, Anaconda, the greatest little city in the world. As long as my heart beats, I will always treasure it."

So dramatic was the surgery that one of the nurses came to my room and directed me that hospital rules required her to ask me, "Do you have depression that leads you to thoughts of suicide?" She almost said it in an apologetic way but assured me that they were required to ask this question of every patient who went through such a traumatic event. Despite being a bit shocked by that, I confidently assured her that I had no thoughts whatsoever of giving up my own life.

While I felt indescribably more weak and void of energy than at any previous point in my life, combined with the physical bodily pain that comes after such a week of death and subsequent major surgery, the reality was that my moment of communing personally with God the Eternal Father and Jesus Christ had continued to have my spirit and soul so lifted and confident that never once did I doubt that one day, in the Lord's own time and as far off as it seemed at that moment, I would be returned to great health and strength—all in His name and for that portion of His work and glory that He still has intended for me to complete.

During the next three to four months, the reality of the depth of my recovery unfolded. I had qualified for early release by completing vital steps of simple exercise and a confident, positive demeanor, which allowed me to be released from the hospital just three days after surgery. I was given many critical medical prescriptions to take daily, but one that I chose not to take was the bottle of painkillers.=" To me, suffering a little pain was a small price to pay for what I had lived through. Physically and spiritually I knew I could overcome all, come what may. However, my second day home made it clear how much of a struggle that would be. With Nancy holding on to me by my side, our instruction was to begin walking at least five minutes a day. While that may not sound challenging, that initial walk a half block up the sidewalk was utterly exhausting to me. I begged Nancy to turn us back so I could go lay down after completing my mandatory hike. As I returned to my couch, my head was spinning and I found I had depleted all of my strength in such a small amount of time.

Never in my life had I experienced anything similar to that kind of exhaustion. While I was proud and joyous to be home again, I struggled mentally with the certainty of the further challenges I now faced. Necessary medications for heart function and cholesterol control, while critical to my recovery, were very new to me and required several long weeks for my mind and body to adjust to. Thanks to the drill sergeant prompting of my sweet companion, I increased the length of my daily strolls each day, and each day I felt the added effects as I triumphantly returned home. My limited walking consisted of short, tempered steps. Each time I glanced in the mirror I felt I was looking at someone else, and in many ways, I was. My weight dropped dramatically, almost fifteen pounds in those first two weeks. The mental portions of my challenges often came late at night, when I would wake up and be taunted by the adversary about impending death. It was overwhelming at times, and I found that constant prayer was essential to overcome it. I even felt it helpful to write down a list of ten reasons why I could and would live through this—which I read and reread often to comfort my natural mind and body. It became painfully clear to me that had I not received that miraculous visitation from the Almighty, I would desperately be toiling in this extremely perilous position alone.

Nevertheless, I *did* have that incredible, miraculous visitation. And each second of each day, as I struggled physically and mentally, that glorious knowledge allowed me to rise above it all.

Coming to life on this earth, I believe, was a divine plan from our Father in heaven to allow each of us an opportunity to reconcile our earthly minds and bodies with our spiritual souls. Accordingly, I did all I could to seek the knowledge of rich blessings in what I was experiencing. I came to know that by the spirit of God alone we can overcome anything. Perhaps my most precious gift during that time came through the scriptures. Every word of God I read or heard was absolute spiritual gold to me. From the very first night after returning home from the hospital, Nancy set up our iPad to verbally read to us from the Bible and *The Book of Mormon*. Without fail, every verse came alive to me and spoke to me of who I was, where I was going, and what I needed to do. I would fight through the rigors of each day and consider those final moments before sleep a great, great reward and strength.

In time, my physical scars began to vanish, including the remnants of the six-inch chest opening that extended vertically over my heart. The months ahead would be filled with heavy doses of body-draining energy through rigorous exercising that pushed me to my limit daily. Many days the anxiety of it all would be nearly unbearable, but knowing that the Lord had promised I would return to health kept me moving toward that goal with confidence and determination. I *knew* I was alive for a purpose, so each minute of the day I pushed on.

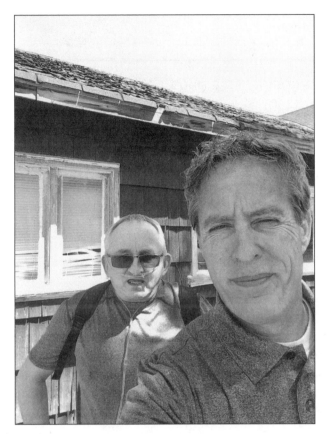

My lifelong friend, Tracy Moses, standing with me in front of
the very house he grew up in some 50 years after we first met.

"In the end, or in this case, what appeared to be the end ~ I
found myself realizing that the one true thing we need to concern ourselves with in life is to learn to walk in the footsteps
of our still living Savior, Jesus Christ. In what was quite nearly
my last hours of life–it was my family and friends like Obe,
Striz and Tracy who rushed to my side from far away places,
along with an overwhelming appreciation and love of the man
who lived so perfectly that we are all able to die and yet live
again, that held importance. My only lingering concern after
visiting those heavenly gates was to make sure that as long
as I live, I will do my best to do things that are pleasing unto
Him, because the day will surely come for all of us to have that
grand and spectacular meeting with Him ~ and joy will be ours
the more "spotless from the world" he finds us.

Eight months later, and to the positive surprise of my doctor, I now feel fully returned to health. I proved it by successfully completing a four-hour hike to Malan's Peak near Ogden, carrying a grandchild a good portion of the way. And when I returned, I played a few games of pickleball. Being alive is a grand blessing, as are each of the precious and additional minutes the Lord is allowing me to spend with my family and friends. I will never forget the day I died, nor the way the Lord wants me to live.

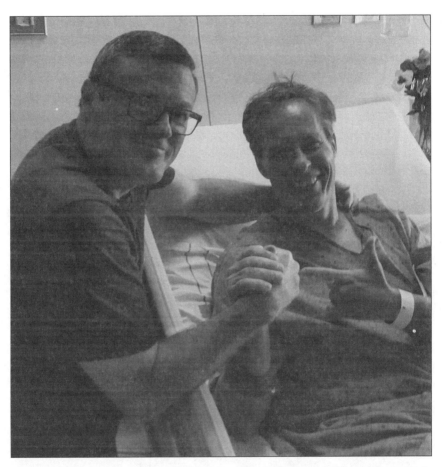

Tom and Pam Oberweiser arrived at McKay Dee Hospital in Ogden, Utah from Billings, Montana just hours after the heart attack. Mike Strizich would arrive a short time later. "I thought I'd seen angels as they walked past my door frantically searching for my hospital room"